FIREBALLS IN MY EUCHARIST

Fight Cancer Smarter

Joseph J. Pinzone, MD, MBA, FACP

Fireballs in My Eucharist: Fight Cancer Smarter
ISBN-978-0-9822943-0-7

For more information visit
www.josephpinzone.com

Published by

Cureiocity
HEALTHCARE LLC

1 2 3 4 5 6 7 8 9 0

TABLE OF CONTENTS

DISCLAIMER

The contents of this book are for informational and educational purposes, and represent my opinions, interpretation and communication of medical information, and not those of any other individual, organization or institution.

This book is not intended to be a substitute for professional medical advice, diagnosis, or treatment. I have made an effort to verify the accuracy of the information, but errors might have inadvertently been included in this book. In addition, medical research and practice is constantly changing; and therefore, some of the information in this book may become obsolete or inaccurate over time. Always seek the advice of your physician or other qualified healthcare provider with any questions that you may have regarding a medical condition or information in this book. The author and publisher expressly disclaim responsibility for any adverse effects arising from the use, reliance on, or application of information in this book.

In this book I deal very openly with many difficult issues relevant to cancer. Therefore, reading this book might engender fear and anxiety, particularly if you have not yet received or had time to deal with a diagnosis of cancer or if you have not yet seen your doctor. However, confronting our fears can often help us to transcend them. Reading this book can help you to become more familiar and comfortable with key medical concepts and issues. Working through some fears before entering the doctor's office might help to lessen anxiety, and allow you to focus your questions during your appointment when you have limited time to build rapport and obtain information. Dealing with anxiety is a good first step to becoming a more effective patient. Claire is a fictional patient, and any reference to her or other medical situations that in any way resembles real persons or situations was entirely unintentional.

Acknowledgements

I want to thank my family, who has been encouraging, patient, and supportive. My wife Lisa always kept me focused and motivated, and she believed in my work to create a better path for people living with cancer. I am also indebted to her because the powerful image of the woman gracing the cover of this book is her artistic work. Our two children, whose zeal and energy recharge my spirit daily, made writing this book that much more meaningful. In them, I find the meaning in my life, as well as the will to live a better life and help others.

Life is fascinating, and patients reflect that wonder in their strength, their desire to live another day and to take advantage of what medicine has to offer, their ability to be unphased, their vulnerability, their quirkiness, their sadness and anger, their quest to feel good, and their ability to inspire those around them. It amazes me how readily and profoundly patients trust doctors with their lives and the lives of their family members. It's what humbles us as doctors and keeps us striving for constant improvement. I want to thank my patients for their trust, and my medical colleagues for their dedication. They are where I found my inspiration to write this book.

I would like to thank my outstanding editor Sherry Wachter for her thoughtful guidance through the process of bringing this book to life and enhancing both its readability and effectiveness. Miriam King, designer extraordinaire, contributed in so many ways. She brought the cover design to a whole new level, formatted the text, drew the illustrations, reviewed the content, and helped www.josephpinzone.com to come to life; and during it all was ever so patient. I would also like to thank Jan Dolph for proofreading this book and offering helpful suggestions and insights.

Finally, I want to thank my colleagues and friends for critical reading of versions of this book, and for their ideas and suggestions. They include: Mark Bloomston, MD; Christine L. Sardo Molmenti, PhD, MPH, RD; Arun Balakumaran, MD, PhD; and Robert Beatey, RN, BSN.

Fireballs in my Eucharist

During my medical training, I evaluated a middle-aged woman whom I had not previously met. I asked her about any past medical problems. She responded, "I have fireballs in my Eucharist." After asking a few more questions, I realized that what she meant to say was: "I have fibroids in my uterus." This encounter touched me deeply. She was my first patient to make this not uncommon mistake; at the time I thought she was unique.

My patient's "fireballs," combined with my later discovery that so many other people don't understand and sometimes can't even pronounce the illness from which they suffer, helped me realize that patient education is critical and can be life-saving, particularly when it comes to the often confusing and complex topic of cancer and its therapy. Educating yourself about your disease, anticipating the mental and physical challenges, learning to better navigate the medical system, and leveraging skill sets that you have developed in other areas of your life just might save your life.

It is not uncommon for patients to get information from family, friends, online, or even people in the doctor's waiting room. These interactions and information can be quite beneficial, but also might be biased or inaccurate. When it comes to understanding your particular disease in order to obtain optimal treatment, your doctor is typically the best person to help you and your family. That's why I wrote this book—to help people with cancer make the most of their doctor visits, communicate accurate information to family and friends, and ultimately make the best healthcare decisions. Your experience with cancer is unique. You need answers tailored to that unique experience. Knowledge truly is power, especially when it means knowing how to acquire the best possible cancer care.

Claire

Meet Claire, a busy 50-year-old executive. She represents no one specific, and yet she is just like any of us. Claire believes in regular medical checkups, but she's a busy woman, and checkups get put off. Finally, though, she makes time to see her family doctor, who recommends that she get a routine **colonoscopy**.* She has no family history of cancer, and dutifully undergoes the procedure. Afterward, the gastroenterologist (a medical specialist in disorders of the digestive tract) who performs the procedure informs her that three small **polyps** were removed and sent for analysis, and that this is not uncommon.

Even through the lingering sedation, Claire senses that this might mean trouble. She waits anxiously for a call regarding the results. After two weeks, Claire finally calls her doctor. The nurse tells her that the doctor will take a look at the **biopsy** results and call her back. The doctor's secretary calls Claire the next day, and asks her to schedule an

*Boldface words are defined in the Glossary at the end of the book.

appointment for the following week. Claire schedules the appointment, then asks the secretary to please just read her the results. The secretary refuses. She explains that she is not allowed to communicate medical information over the phone, and that the doctor has specifically asked that Claire come in to review the results.

Now Claire is worried. She immediately logs onto the Internet and Googles "colon cancer." She is overwhelmed when her search results in 25 million hits, but she spends a little time clicking and reading online, and she concludes that the vast majority of polyps found during a colonoscopy are **benign**. She logs off and breathes a little easier.

The following week Claire shows up at the gastroenterologist's office alone. Her husband plans on going with her until they remember that he needs to take their daughter to an SAT prep class. The nurse shows Claire into an examination room right on schedule. By the time the doctor comes in fifteen minutes later, Claire's stomach is in knots. The doctor tells her one of the **lesions** he removed during the colonoscopy is cancerous.

"I don't understand," Claire says. "Can you repeat that? I'm not sure I heard you correctly."

"I'm sorry to have to tell you that, but of course that's why we do these tests," the doctor responds.

Claire's mind goes blank. She hears very little of what the doctor says after that, but she still nods politely. The gastroenterologist tells her to ask her family doctor for a referral to a surgeon, but Claire hasn't really understood anything since the doctor told her she had cancer. She thanks the doctor, leaves the office, gets in her car—and ends up missing the freeway exit to her neighborhood. She takes the next one, thinking she'll turn around and go home. At the bottom of the exit ramp she sees a fast food drive-thru. She pulls in, orders a coffee, tries to call her husband, and ends up calling her secretary instead. This is not good. And Claire has a feeling things are about to get a lot worse.

～

While nothing Claire might have done would have made her **diagnosis** easy to hear, there are a number of things she might have done differently to make it easier to manage. How might Claire have set herself up for a more effective interaction with her gastroenterologist? How might she have handled his instructions about calling her doctor for a referral? Is there a way her family could have been more involved in her initial care? How should Claire communicate with and involve her family at this point and as she enters treatment?

When we speak of the "world of medicine," we mean exactly that. Medicine is a world with a language and customs all its own—a world in which learning to speak the language and understand the customs can literally be a life-or-death matter. Think of this as your guidebook. We'll discuss ways you can frame the key issues and questions to make your dealings with the world of medicine, and particularly medical providers, more intuitive, effective, and reassuring. We'll demystify the medical system, and reinforce your awareness of and reliance on resources and skills you already have in order to get the best medical care. This book doesn't promise less work for you, just a road map for navigating the world of medicine efficiently and effectively.

Learn the Language: The first step in understanding a complex topic like modern medical care is knowing the language. Throughout the text, words in bold are defined in the glossary at the end of this book. In addition, the glossary contains other terms that do not appear in the text. You can refer to the glossary as needed while reading this book. You might also find it valuable to read the glossary from beginning to end as a separate chapter to reinforce what you learned.

Plan Ahead: Take time to organize your thoughts before every interaction with the medical system, just as you would for any other important meeting. Often patients don't know exactly why they have come to see a particular doctor or are having a certain test. Preparation might include learning and reviewing information, organizing and rehearsing questions, and getting yourself into the right frame of mind.

First impressions are important. Creating an open, honest, intelligent dialogue with your doctor starts with your first medical visit. Your doctor's job is to interview and examine you in order to help you. But that process works best when you engage and interview the doctor in return. This book will help you craft succinct, informative responses to your doctor's questions and also ask your doctor the right questions. Being well prepared helps your doctor help you, and it makes you a more memorable patient—in a good way. Being memorable for the right reasons can result in more powerful office visits and better healthcare all around.

I've provided some trustworthy resources, but I encourage you to seek out resources beyond those presented in this book. There are multiple perspectives on therapies and **clinical trials** that might be appropriate for your condition. The good news is you are likely already quite effective at finding information and resources, and we'll look at ways to hone and polish those skills in the world of medicine. The research you do on your own, whether online or by talking with people, can be a powerful tool, but always discuss your findings with your doctor so you can make the vital decisions about your health together.

Work with your loved ones as well as your doctors as you face the challenge of managing your illness. This book outlines strategies for including friends and family members in your care. In addition, you may be able to find camaraderie and companionship through cancer support organizations, some of which are listed later in this book. Finally, professional help from a counselor, psychologist, or psychiatrist might be essential in helping you work through illness-related issues—and help you manage your illness and your life more effectively. Your doctor can probably provide you with a referral.

I wrote this book as though you, the reader, are the patient with cancer; but of course you might be a loved one of a patient, a caregiver, or a medical professional. Perhaps you simply want to learn more about cancer or how to navigate the healthcare system. In order to keep my writing brief and readable, I sometimes discuss techniques or ways to improve your effectiveness as a patient very succinctly. Not every suggestion will be feasible in every circumstance. However, if you find any of this information valuable and can put it into action, my mission has been accomplished. As a physician, I know that at times my writing might sound "clinical"—that is to say, less than personal. If you find this to be the case, please accept my apologies. It is with these thoughts in mind that I offer you this book. I hope you find it valuable and that it serves you well.

NOTES

CHAPTER 1

Cancer Explained

Understanding what cancer is, how it forms in the body, and what issues might arise in dealing with it is key to any therapeutic decisions you and your care team will make. However, cancer is a complex disease. You might want to read this chapter more than once, and make a list of questions to ask your doctor, who will be able to more fully explain the concepts relevant to you.

Our bodies are made up of trillions of **cells,** the basic building blocks of life (see **Figure 1**). Cells that comprise one organ look and function differently than cells from other organs. Liver cells are different from heart cells, which are different from brain cells. So what makes each type of cell different? The answer is a bit complex and requires some background information. All cells in our bodies have the same **deoxyribonucleic acid (DNA)**, except for sperm and egg cells, which have only half the DNA. DNA resides in the nucleus (control center) of cells, and it is simply a string of four different

Figure 1. Normal vs. Cancer Cells

Normal Cells

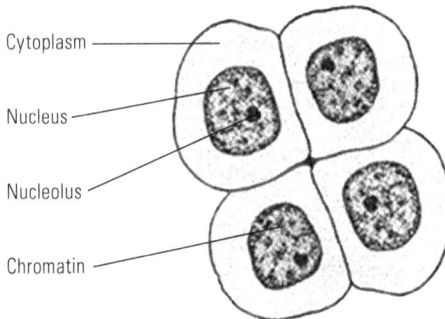

Normal Cells: Lots of cytoplasm relative to the size of the nucleus. Single nucleus with small amount of chromatin (DNA bound to proteins). Regular cell border with all cells in contact with each other (except for some cell types like normal blood cells).

Cancer Cells

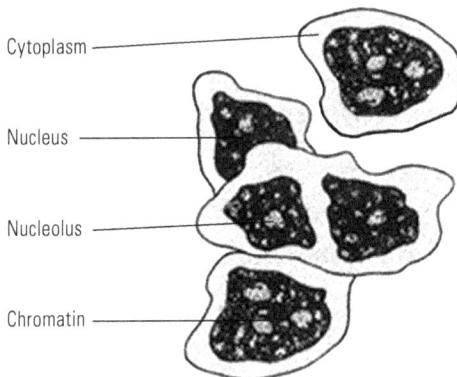

Cancer Cells: Less cytoplasm relative to the size of the nucleus. Cells typically have lots of chromatin, and can have one nucleus or more than one (nucleoli). Irregular cell borders often occur, with some cells breaking off and traveling through the lymph system and/or bloodstream to grow in other parts of the body (metastasize).

chemical compounds (adenine, cytosine, thymine, and guanine) called bases that are typically represented as A, C, T, G (see **Figure 2**). Each cell contains twenty-three pairs of **chromosomes** made up of DNA that is millions of bases long. (Again, sperm and eggs have half the DNA because they have twenty-three chromosomes, not twenty-three pairs.) The specific sequence of bases in a stretch of DNA provides the code for a **gene.** The number of bases comprising different genes vary from just a few to thousands. Each gene has a unique sequence of bases, and each cell contains approximately 20,000 genes.

Most genes hold the code for making **protein.** Proteins are made up of chemical building blocks called amino acids. The specific sequence of bases that makes up a gene provides the blueprint our cellular machinery uses to assemble the amino acids into a unique protein. The unique sequence of bases in each of the 20,000 genes correlates directly with the unique sequence of the resultant protein. In fact, our cells can produce more that 20,000 different proteins because of different ways the DNA sequences can be read. Though cells are made up of many substances, proteins are the basic building blocks.

Different proteins function in different ways within each cell. Some proteins give the cell structure, whereas other proteins are involved in doing the business of the cells. For instance, many proteins within breast cells are involved in the production of milk, which contains other types of protein that serve as an important source of nutrition for a baby.

So what accounts for the differences between cells? Cells are choosy; they don't use all 20,000 of the genes they contain to produce proteins. To illustrate the point, I have created the following fictitious scenario. A liver cell might use 10,000 genes to code for 12,000 different proteins, whereas a heart cell might use 9,000 genes (5,000 of the same genes the liver cell uses and 4,000 other ones) to code for 14,000 different proteins. The specific subset of genes each cell uses produces a unique complement of proteins. The unique proteins within each type of cell work together to create distinct cells designed for different functions. Having one set of proteins results in rounded cells that detoxify our blood and process nutrients (liver cells), whereas having a different set of proteins results in long muscle cells that contract (heart cells).

Cancer occurs in our cells as they multiply during their normal life cycle. Data now suggests that all organs in the body can regenerate to some degree. Each organ in our body is made up mostly of mature cells that carry out the functioning of that organ. However, each organ has a small number of cells

Figure 2. Metabolism of Normal vs. Cancer Cells

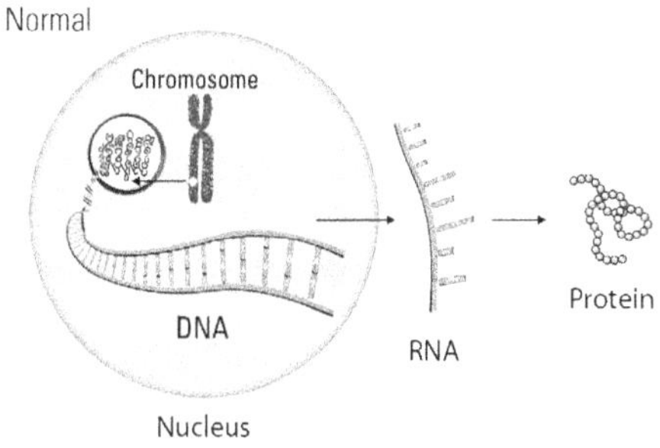

Normal

Chromosome / DNA / RNA / Protein / Nucleus

Normal Cells: Chromosomes, located in the cell nucleus, contain DNA. DNA is composed of "bases— adenine, guanine, cytosine and thymidine (abbreviated A, C, T, G)—linked to one another in a string or ladder. Each chromosome contains millions of bases strung together in a very specific sequence. The sequence varies, though very little in terms of percentage, from human to human. Some of those strings of bases "code" for genes (each chromosome has hundreds to thousands of genes, with about 20,000 total genes in our genome), while some are non-coding bases (that is, they are not part of a gene sequence). The non-coding bases are also important as they connect genes and/or regulate gene expression. Genes are then transcribed into messenger RNA (mRNA), which is exported from the nucleus and translated into protein. One gene can code for one or more proteins.

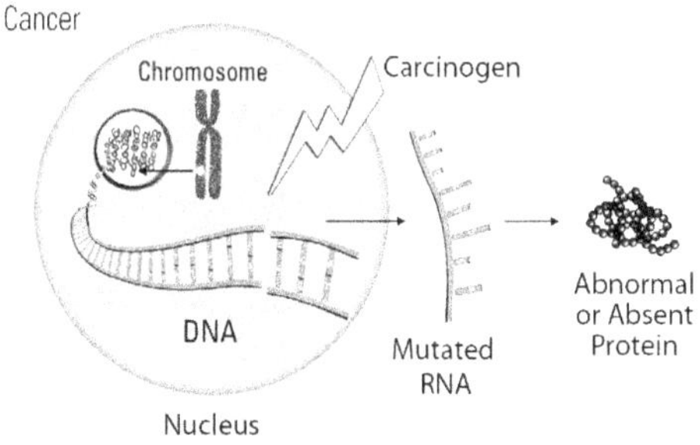

Cancer

Chromosome / Carcinogen / DNA / Mutated RNA / Abnormal or Absent Protein / Nucleus

Cancer Cells: The DNA in the chromosomes of cancer cells has been damaged (mutated) in some way by a carcinogen—a cancer-causing agent or event such as UV light, radiation, toxins in tobacco, etc.—or is mutated by chance as cells divide. If the DNA is mutated, the mRNA and resultant proteins (typically those involved in cell growth) are absent or abnormal. It usually takes multiple key mutations in a given cell to "cause" cancer. Some people are born with one or more mutations in a given cell type, or in all their cells, that make it more likely that they will develop cancer, though they typically need other mutations as well. The incidence of most cancers increases with age as mutations accrue over time. Since the mutated, dysfunctional proteins result in a growth advantage of cancer cells over normal cells, the cancer cells can grow faster and/or live longer than normal cells. This can lead to even more mutations, which is why some cancers can become more aggressive over time.

called **stem cells.** In children and adults, the stem cells of a particular organ are responsible for making more of that organ to replace cells that die naturally. These are called somatic stem cells. Somatic stem cells are different from fetal stem cells, which create organs as the fetus matures in the womb. While somatic stem cells repair and replace cells as they die naturally, in some situations where many cells die—such as heart attacks—cells are not replaced.

Skin provides a good example of how the normal cellular life cycle works (see **Figure 3**). Mature skin cells protect us, and as skin cells die or are shed they need to be replaced. For example, if you get sunburned, the top layers of your skin peel off, and you need to make more skin to replace what was lost. There is a layer of skin stem cells below the surface of your skin that divides to make more skin cells. When skin stem cells divide they produce offspring cells. The offspring cells are slightly different from the parent stem cells, and end up with characteristics that make them a bit more like mature skin cells. The offspring cells then divide to produce their own offspring cells that are even more like mature skin cells. This process continues for several rounds of cell division until the offspring cells gradually acquire all the features of mature skin cells. Mature skin cells are unable to divide further.

Now consider the fact that the sun's ultraviolet (UV) rays are able to penetrate skin and hit less mature skin cells, including stem cells, which have the ability to divide. The UV rays cause **mutations** (damage) in the DNA of these cells or even damage an entire chromosome. The damaged part of the cells' DNA might encode a specific gene or control whether a gene is expressed into a protein. Cells can repair many of the DNA breaks. However, if a cell is unable to repair certain mutations, then the damaged gene in that cell begins to produce fewer, more, or abnormal proteins, depending on the specific mutation. The resultant protein changes can cause future cell divisions to occur less efficiently, in which case the cells die before they become mature skin cells. However, sometimes the protein problems cause the cells to divide *more* efficiently or to become resistant to cell death. These abnormal cells can then grow and divide to form a **tumor,** which may or may not be cancerous. In addition to specific causative factors such as UV light, mutations can occur randomly during cell division. To make matters worse, some tumor cells can actually acquire mutations more rapidly than normal cells. That's why some cancers become more aggressive as time goes by.

A tumor that stays in its original location without spreading is a **benign** tumor. Benign tumors can

Figure 3.

Normal Maturation of Skin Cells vs. How Skin Cancer Forms

All cells in our body have somatic stem cells, which replenish cells that die in the normal course of our lives. However, sometimes when large areas of certain organs die, such as happens in a heart attack, all the cells cannot be replaced by stem cells. In contrast, one can have a large area of the liver removed and it will typically regenerate. For some tissues, such as skin, the process of replenishing cells tends to be a more rapid occurrence because we lose lots of skin cells every day.

Normal

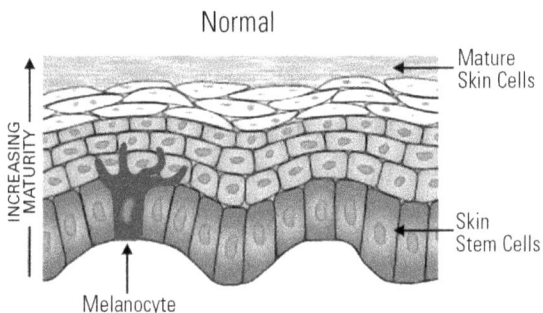

Normal Skin: Maturation of skin cells occurs as the stem cells, located at the deepest layers of the skin, divide. As they divide, the cells that are produced move closer to the surface of the skin; as this happens the cells acquire more characteristics of mature skin cells, and lose their ability to divide.

Skin Cancer

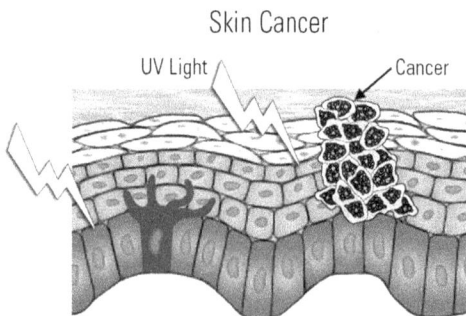

Skin Cancer: When our skin cells are exposed to carcinogens, the most well-known and pervasive one being UV light from the sun, DNA mutations resulting in either absent or abnormal DNA and RNA (and ultimately absent or dysfunctional proteins) results. The current theory is that the more immature the cell is when it accrues the key cancer-causing mutations, the more aggressive the cancer is, though this is not proven. If the theory is correct, UV light that causes cancer in skin stem cells results in a more aggressive cancer than if a more mature skin cell with less replicative potential were adversely affected by UV light.

still do damage as they grow, but they do not spread to other organs. However, if the cells have the ability to detach from the original tumor, travel through the blood or other body fluids, and invade and grow somewhere else in the body (**metastasize**), then that tumor is **malignant** (cancerous). No matter what organ the cells attach themselves to, the site of the original tumor defines the type of cancer. For example, if a person develops colon cancer that metastasizes to the liver, the person has metastatic colon cancer, not colon cancer and liver cancer.

Cancer can develop in many different organs of the body, and there are approximately 200 types of cancer. The same type of cancer, and even the same subtype, can behave quite differently in different people. Because mutations occur in stem cells or other cells as they divide to help replenish our lost cells, tissues and organs that replenish themselves more quickly tend to form cancers at a higher rate. That's one reason why skin, lung, and colon cancers are so common. These cells are all exposed to the "outside" of your body and/or come in contact with toxins. Skin cells are exposed to the sun; lung cells are exposed to air pollution and cigarette smoke; and colon cells are exposed to any toxic substances we might ingest. However, cancer can also occur commonly is some organs that are not directly exposed to the external environment.

Many things in the environment, such as UV rays, tobacco smoke, or radiation can cause DNA breaks that lead to cancer. However, some people are born with a specific mutation in a particular gene. The mutation can be inherited (passed down from a parent) or spontaneous (occurring in the patient, but not in a parent). When someone is born with a specific mutation in their DNA, the resultant abnormal gene is present in all cells of the body. In some cases, the mutation can result in the production of an abnormal protein that can lead to non-cancerous diseases such as Tay-Sachs disease or sickle cell anemia. However, in other cases, the abnormal protein gives cells in a certain organ a growth advantage, which can make cancer more likely to occur there.

Our immune systems provide an important defense against many cancers as well as infection. However, cancer cells often evade detection by our immune systems and, in some cases, use immune cells to help the cancer cells grow. Recently we have begun to understand these processes better, and we are now exploring and using immune-based anti-cancer therapies to treat some types of cancer.

NOTES

NOTES

12

CHAPTER 2

Build and Lead Your Medical Team

A personal medical team composed of loved ones, doctors, and other medical personnel all working together can be invaluable. Typically, the best person to lead that team is you, the patient. Like a successful business, a successful medical team is made up of people who are passionate about serving others' needs, and who clearly define and achieve goals. Obviously, your medical team needs to be passionate about helping you, but how do you ensure that passion is present in all your team members at all times? Even though they all might care about you, sometimes it can be challenging to motivate your team. Similarly, setting clear goals makes good sense, while the path to reaching those goals might be less self-evident.

Using a business model to manage your health-care may seem odd. Business terms and concepts are unfamiliar to many of us (I will define key terms and concepts as we go along). Also, some companies' recent questionable and, in certain cases, criminal behavior may make the thought of applying business principles to your personal medical care unappealing. But here's the thing: Like healthcare at its best, business at its best meets the needs of all involved parties openly, honestly, and fairly and, like people everywhere, the vast majority of those who engage in business are good caring folks trying to do the right thing. Your doctor and hospital are engaged in the business of delivering healthcare, and typically the best healthcare providers and institutions are financially healthy themselves. Assuming that this makes sense to you, let's consider the structure of your team.

Your team operates in the service sector, and the main service your team provides is high-quality, compassionate healthcare (to you!). You will function as both your team's leader and main customer. Other customers might include your family members and anyone else who is invested in your well-being. Balancing the roles of "leader" and "customer" can sometimes be a bit tricky. To build and manage your team, you must address three processes:

1. Get the right people in the right jobs.
2. Construct a winning strategy.
3. Put your strategy into action!

It is usually best if the leader (typically this is you) functions as the Chairman of the Board & Chief Executive Officer (CEO). This means that you can and should delegate various tasks. Ultimately, though, you are responsible for everything related to your health-care. You do the hiring and firing, you make the final decision on strategy, and you see that the work gets done. Being both the CEO and the customer can be a bit confusing; but the dual role brings with it a huge advantage—the CEO can instantly act on customer feedback.

Many people with cancer benefit from having a **care partner**. This might be a loved one or friend. Using the business analogy, your care partner would function as the Vice Chairman. The Vice Chairman helps you to oversee the team strategy, functions as a sounding board for you, and helps with high-level decision-making.

Your main cancer doctor (potentially a **medical oncologist**) will be the Chief Operating Officer (COO). The COO will help you to set your strategy and, more importantly, help you define and implement the tactics to accomplish that strategy. In other words, the COO might help you set goals, determine next steps, and find and hire the right people—the other doctors involved in your care—to get the job done.

There might be overlap in how your care partner and doctors serve you. At successful companies, each member's skill set defines that person's role and contribution as much as his or her official job description.

For example, your care partner might also be a medical practitioner who can help find the best physicians for you. The business framework is the starting point from which you go on to organize your healthcare team in the way that is most effective for you.

You may want to designate a Chief Financial Officer (CFO) to deal with the revenue (the money from your insurance company, your household income, or savings) needed to pay for your services and goods. The CFO can be you, your spouse, or your care partner, but it is typically best to have one or, at most, two people take final responsibility. Otherwise, your enterprise might not get reimbursed as it should, which could impede team progress.

You will also need consultants—other doctors who will be responsible for providing opinions or carrying out specific functions. Consultants might include the **surgical oncologist** who performs surgery to try to remove a tumor or the **radiation oncologist** who administers radiation treatments. Though the surgeon and radiation oncologist might treat you, one of them might or might not function as your main cancer doctor, depending on variations among institutions and geographic regions, as well as your specific circumstances.

In some cases, a doctor with a completely different specialty might serve as your main doctor.

People with thyroid cancer, for instance, might have an endocrinologist (a physician who takes care of patients with hormone issues such as diabetes and thyroid problems) as their main cancer doctor.

Your nurse or nurses—your customer care managers, in business terms—are key team members. Nurses are a vital resource; they help implement your **care plan**. They often administer treatments, keep you safe and comfortable, and provide and relay information. Without them your entire medical plan, as well as the relationship between you and your doctor can fall apart. Oncology nurses, who administer **chemotherapy**, assess your clinical status, and often spend much more time with patients than do doctors, typically have advanced training.

Nurses can suggest therapies to address **symptoms** such as pain and medication side effects, catch medication errors, help coordinate care, and help with the patient's emotional needs. Nurse practitioners (NPs) and physician assistants (PAs) have more advanced clinical training. NPs and PAs often practice under the direct supervision of a physician and can be part of more complex procedures and decision-making than nurses.

Just like in a company, the administrative staff members of your healthcare team—appointment schedulers and billing personnel at doctors' offices or hospitals—are key team members and can be helpful patient advocates. They can help you to make that key connection to other doctors, get tests or treatments ordered sooner, or get properly reimbursed by insurance companies. Administrative staff members often have experience and know tricks of the trade that can help you cut through layers of bureaucracy. If you are able to develop a rapport with a particular individual at your insurance company, then he or she can be a critical part of your team as well. Finally, there might be other jobs within your healthcare team that you will need to fill given your particular circumstances.

Once you've got the right people in the right jobs, it becomes critical to get their attention and motivate them. This is exactly what you need to do to make a business successful, and only the best business leaders are able to do this consistently. If anyone proves to be difficult to deal with, treat him or her dispassionately and work around that person as you would in business. In some cases you might need to "fire" a team member. Remember, it's you…your body, your time, and your money that are most important. Success here can improve the quality and maybe even the quantity of your life.

Communication and Organization are Key

Communication and organization are key to managing your medical care, just as in business. Combined with systematic documentation, good communication keeps your team moving in the right direction, giving you a way to hold people accountable. Your system doesn't have to be elaborate, but it does have to be well-organized and consistent—and it needs to be based on solid, accurate information.

The golden rule: First seek to understand, then seek to be understood. Asking questions is as important as any treatment, because the answers you receive will guide you to the right treatment decisions for you. Your doctor should help you to become informed so that you can decide what is right for you. However, some doctors are better at this than others. It is your responsibility to make sure your doctor provides you with the knowledge you need.

Visits with your doctor are like strategy meetings at work. There should be open-ended discussion, but everyone should also come to the table with specific thoughts written down as a starting point from which to work. Before your first meeting with a doctor or healthcare professional, determine your priorities and prepare a list of questions based on them.

At the completion of the meeting, everyone should walk away with a written plan of action (POA). *Note that you or your care partner will probably be the ones writing that plan, as your doctor might not provide a written assessment of what transpired during the visit.*

A POA is simply an outline of next steps, and the tasks necessary to make those steps happen. For each task, note the name of the person responsible for the task, a timeline for when the task (or the steps in the task) should be completed, and the date you can contact that person and expect to hear the results. Keep a running log somewhere—in your planner, on your laptop, wherever works for you. Remember to write down specific dates for chemotherapy sessions, surgery, and/or diagnostic tests.

Note in chronological order exactly what needs to get done and who is responsible for each action. Write down names of your healthcare providers and their role so you don't forget them, and so that you can hold people accountable. If you use this simple system, you might end up more organized than your doctor. In fact, sending a copy of this list to your doctor is a good practice to "close the loop" after your visit.

For example, you can write:

MARCH **2**	Visit with Dr. "Medical Oncologist". After visit, get blood drawn and pick up prescription for "medication A."
MARCH **3**	Call Dr. "Radiation Oncologist" to set up an appointment for evaluation to determine whether external beam radiation therapy is appropriate. Then call Dr. "Medical Oncologist's" office to let her know the appointment date.
TBD	Dr. "Medical Oncologist" will call Dr. "Radiation Oncologist" to discuss my case within one week of that appointment and will then call me. If I do not hear from Dr. "Medical Oncologist" in that timeframe I will call her.
MARCH **9**	Call Dr. "Medical Oncologist's" office to obtain blood work results from March 2 visit—I plan to speak with the nurse, but will ask to speak with the doctor if the results are abnormal.
APRIL **1**	April 1 – Next appointment with Dr. "Medical Oncologist"

The Patient-Doctor Relationship

Choosing the best care for you

Doctors come in all shapes, sizes, personalities, and specialties. How do you choose the best doctor for you? A doctor who focuses his or her career on treating a very specific ailment, particularly if it is a rare disease, might be regarded as "the best," but there are no medical Olympics, competitions, or ratings systems that pit doctors against each other to determine skills. Realistically speaking, there is no way to determine which one doctor is the best.

Even if we could, the likelihood of that doctor being close by is astronomically small. Part of determining which doctor is best for you is proximity and availability. Should you travel 2,000 miles and recover from your surgery away from family and friends to get to the best colorectal surgeon to remove a comparatively common colon cancer that you've caught at the earliest, most curable stage? Perhaps not. On the other hand, if you have a rare cancer and there are only three surgeons in the world who can remove your tumor and cure you, buy a plane ticket!

For the vast majority of conditions, you can determine, with a reasonable degree of certainty, the *optimal* doctor to see. *Optimal,* as opposed to *best,* means that the doctor is both competent and passionate about caring for you—and that reaching him or her for treatment will not unduly deplete you and your family's much-needed time, money, and mental and physical energy.

Once you've identified your optimal doctor, forming a healthy doctor-patient relationship is key. What does a healthy doctor-patient relationship look like? Many people have had nothing but positive relationships with doctors, and that's great—but it's not always the case.

As with any business, customer needs are not always met. Cancer treatment often requires intense interactions with many different doctors and their staff. Choosing a doctor with whom you are comfortable and then putting him or her in charge of your medical care is the first item of business. Knowing how to make your appointments with all of the doctors involved in your treatment as productive and pleasant as possible is the second.

Determining which doctor will be the point person for each specific disease or problem is essential. Do not count on your family doctor to do this without your input. He or she may be able to offer you information about various specialists, but only you can choose the doctor with whom you feel most comfortable. And once you've made that choice, be sure to communicate your decision clearly to everyone involved. Not doing so can result in confusion, miscommunication, and potentially even errors.

Any doctor you are considering to lead your healthcare team should welcome an interview about his or her experience and comfort level in handling your specific condition. But keep in mind that doctors are people and, therefore, have egos...sometimes big ones!

It makes sense to be respectful of a doctor's dedication and expertise, but when you ask your questions, watch his or her responses closely. If the doctor is incensed, outraged, or dismissive of your questions, this is a big red flag. Obviously, your doctor should have a deep sense of confidence in his or her own abilities, and a slight hint of arrogance is not necessarily a negative. However, significant arrogance is borne out of insecurity and can be dangerous.

The bottom line is that you should be earnest and genuine in your approach to seeking the best care, and you should get a genuine, caring answer in response. When a patient asks me whether I am the right doctor to treat a particular disease, I answer them honestly. If I think that one of my patients would be better served by a different physician, I generally suggest this before the patient raises the question.

If a patient asks me if he or she should get a second opinion, I typically say that two heads can often be better than one. However, I also probe to see exactly why *they* think they might need more advice, so I can make sure I am serving their needs.

It goes without saying that doctors should work in the best interest of their patients. Chances are your doctor is doing that, but there are many intangibles that go into creating that all-important feeling of trust and confidence you want to have in your doctor. Is there a great "fit" between you (your personality, your medical condition, etc.) and your doctor (personality, area of expertise, etc.)? If not, get a second opinion, or switch doctors.

Get the right referrals

With the exception of your care partner, you will be hiring your medical team members, including your doctors. Choosing your doctor first usually makes the most sense. Sometimes this will be your main cancer doctor, but if you do not yet have a diagnosis, the doctor who makes the diagnosis might not be your main cancer physician.

While it is important to choose team members who are both competent and passionate about your recovery, each position on the team will require different skills and personality traits. However, for all roles you need basic qualities such as integrity (the person needs to be honest with him or herself and with you). In addition, you want every person on your team to treat you and others with respect, and have outstanding knowledge and competence. But two of the most important qualities that are needed are sometimes never critically assessed. First, you want each team member to be passionate about his or her work. Second, each person needs to have a track record of efficient follow-through on tasks.

Much has been written on the topic of how to get a good referral. In the business world, companies will often look close to home first. Many consultants are hired from among a tightly networked circle of candidates. These professionals have trusted names in the industry in general, and they may have served others who work for or are familiar with the company.

In hiring for your healthcare team, look first to trusted entities. Many of the best doctors come from institutions with the best reputations, though sometimes smaller, less-known organizations have doctors with outstanding reputations and abilities as well.

Family, friends and acquaintances whose judgment you trust can be valuable referral sources. However, they may not assess their doctors in the same ways you would, so be sure to ask your own questions, rather than hiring a healthcare provider based on a referral alone.

Start with the criteria listed below, add any other qualities you are looking for, and rate your doctor. Base your rating on your own perceptions when meeting with a potential doctor, as well as on input from trusted people who have had experience with this physician. You might only need to visit one doctor, but if you feel more comfortable visiting others, then do so. If your first two or three visits don't even come close to matching your criteria, either you are not generating your short list effectively, or you're in an area that has a shortage of good physicians.

Rate each quality below on a scale from 1 to 5, with 1 the lowest rating and 5 the highest.

_____ Integrity

_____ Compassion

_____ Professionalism/respect

_____ Unrushed manner

_____ Service/responsiveness

_____ Competence

_____ Positive energy

_____ Passion

_____ Ability to get things done

_____ "Gut feeling" that this is the optimal doctor for me

Definitions

Integrity – Do you feel that this doctor is honest and forthright?

Compassion – Do you feel that this doctor cares about you?

Professionalism – Did this doctor demonstrate a professional manner?

Respect – Did you feel like your opinion mattered during the conversation?

Unrushed manner – Did you feel that there was enough time allotted for your visit?

Service – Was the pre- and post-visit experience with the doctor and staff pleasant?

Responsiveness – Were the doctor and staff courteous and prompt in answering calls?

Competence – Did this doctor have a well-reasoned thought process regarding your diagnosis, prognosis, and treatment plan, and was this based on current evidence? Did he or she communicate the proposed plan to you clearly and confirm that you understood everything? Does your doctor run clinical trials (this often reflects a higher degree of specialization and expertise)? Is he or she a member of professional organizations?

Positive energy – Did this doctor light up the room? Though not always essential, if backed by competence, this attribute can promote a more pleasant, approachable, and comfortable environment and experience.

Passion – Does this doctor want you to feel better as much as you do? Is it obvious that this doctor loves what he or she does? This attribute is essential.

Ability to get things done – Did this doctor or office facilitate the completion of your treatment plan and anticipate and avoid logistical, insurance, or other roadblocks? Did he or she clarify who was going to do which task (schedule appointments with other doctors or follow up on diagnostic tests, etc.) you, the doctor, the nurse, or the administrative assistant? Did the doctor and their office then deliver on their part?

"Gut Feeling" – Do you feel that this is the right doctor to diagnose/treat you?

Usually when a patient goes to see a doctor, the office and/or hospital staff comes with the deal. However, if you find the right doctor for you, but are not satisfied with a particular member of the staff, often another person can be assigned to care for you. Patients and their families often worry that complaining about anything, including staff members, may compromise the care they receive. Sometimes this happens, but fortunately it is not common, particularly if the issue is addressed early.

You might feel vulnerable because medical personnel and their staff seem to have more power than patients and their families. Even though you are paying them, you might feel that you need your doctor and their staff more than they need you. Bear in mind, though, that you hold key powers that balance things out. You can:

1. Walk away and find another practitioner.
2. Give that medical practitioner a bad review (verbally or in writing).
3. Complain to hospital or practice administration (verbally or in writing).
4. Pursue legal action against your doctor.

Doctors understand this, and their desire to truly be kind and help others, stay in business, and avoid conflict and litigation is usually enough to keep the experience pleasant, but not always. In the course of my life I have myself had to walk away from a doctor I didn't connect with, give a doctor a bad review verbally, and even verbally complain about a doctor or staff member. Putting those complaints into writing or litigation is definitely more serious and can usually be avoided. The key to avoiding intense conflict is to determine for each lapse in competence or compassion whether it is important to voice your concern. If so, address the situation quickly and calmly. Be specific. Let the doctor know how you would like to see this issue resolved, or ask their opinion about the best course of action.

Let's go through a few scenarios. I have occasionally encountered a rude person on the other end of the phone when scheduling an appointment with a doctor. Reasons for rudeness vary, but the consequences for the patient can range from anger and frustration to delayed or improper care.

When I encounter a rude person on the telephone, I explain that I am a colleague of the doctor, which usually, but not always, corrects the situation. Most patients will not have this option, and it is just not practical to eliminate every doctor who has an annoying or dysfunctional front desk person. Unless you think the behavior is egregious, in which case I would consider finding another practice, I suggest relying on a few techniques.

Try using your charm and humor to diffuse the situation. If that doesn't work, remind the person that you are ill and need kindness. This will usually disarm him or her and you might even make a friend.

If these things do not work, feel free to let the doctor know. If there is a concern about reprisal, just talk to the doctor about it and ask that he or she deal with the situation discreetly. This is an opportunity to see how the doctor deals with conflict, your concerns, and getting things done on your behalf.

When you discuss this with the doctor, be specific about the offending action. You might say something like: "I have had two negative interactions with [name] on your staff, and this is specifically what happened…. Could you please designate someone else to help me with [the function of that person] in the future?"

You should be treated with kindness, compassion and respect

As a group, doctors happen to be some of the nicest, brightest, and most caring folks I know, but still, they and their staff are just people. Remember, they do not know you when you first meet them. It's your job to make a great first impression on them, and it's their job to do the same for you. From the minute I call a doctor's office I expect there to be mutual respect. Your doctor should care about you and you should feel that caring during and after the visit. In addition, your doctor should bring respect and empathy to each visit.

If your doctor is late for your appointment, he or she should apologize. But please realize that sometimes he or she is not totally aware of what time your visit was scheduled. Yes, it's the doctor's job to know that information and be on time, but the interaction with the previous patient may have been complicated and time-consuming, and your doctor is simply trying to juggle a challenging day.

Repeated lateness, of course, signals a systems problem with the way the office schedules patients.

Feel free to point that out and ask that in the future, if the doctor will be late, to please have the staff give you a heads-up and an estimated time of arrival. Finally, your doctor should either exhibit an unhurried manner or acknowledge that he or she is short on time because of an emergency or other situation. In that case, he or she should ensure that in the near future you will have the time together that you need.

The doctor and staff should recognize that you are ill, and that the stress of your illness may be expressed in various ways. They should cut you some slack, and on occasion your healthcare team might be even more understanding than your family or friends.

But if a patient is repeatedly rude and demanding, the doctor and staff will get frustrated or even angry, though they might not show it. Even great doctors and staff members have bad days. It is helpful if the patient is understanding as well. That said, there are several things that are just plain unacceptable from either side of this relationship.

Condescending or contemptuous behavior or threats of any kind have no place in any relationship, particularly the doctor-patient relationship. Also, as in other areas of life, if either party is not truthful, then the relationship cannot proceed in a healthy fashion.

Some doctors simply do not have a great bedside manner; they seem unable to demonstrate significant respect or empathy, or they can't communicate clearly. And, in fact, some doctors (though in my experience very few) are just not nice people. However, the medical school admissions process and the intense experience of medical school and post-graduate training actually do select for really wonderful people in general, and that goes for nurses and other staff as well. These people are there to serve you, and that is usually the way they look at it. If you encounter a doctor with a poor bedside manner, you might consider tolerating *some* shortcomings if the physician is uniquely talented, especially if you do not need to spend much time together.

Get your treatment team to give you the best care

Take control of your relationship with your doctor by being prepared and engaged. It has been said that what children really want is not for their parents to do everything perfectly, but rather for them to be engaged *with* them in their journey through life, to celebrate in victory, and fight the good fight when things are tough. Participation like this takes time and commitment.

This is precisely what most patients want from their doctors—and often what their doctors want from them! Think about it—a doctor is a busy professional with only so much time. He or she cannot teach people basic life skills. Realistically, a doctor can work with whoever comes through the door only to the best of the physician's ability and the ability of the patient.

Your doctor strives for a sense that he or she has helped you and your family. When you feel you have been helped, you can make your doctor's job more fulfilling by demonstrating your gratitude and expressing your thanks. As a bonus, your doctor might work a bit harder and smarter in the quest to help you.

You can trust your doctor's opinion…probably

We've all heard faulty diagnosis stories: A patient with "six months to live" is still alive and healthy 25 years later; or the patient whose "inoperable" tumor is successfully removed by a second doctor. So just how far can you trust your doctor's opinion?

Since knowing this might be a matter of life and death for you, it's important to know that the person you are trusting with your medical care is up to the responsibility. How well your doctor listens to what you have to say, and how your doctor deals with uncertainty can be important indicators. There is no way for you (or your doctor) to be 100 percent certain about anything. Any therapeutic plan that you discuss might or might not work as planned, and it will potentially have adverse effects.

Your doctor should not speak in absolute terms, but neither should he or she fail to give you an opinion. I believe that when some doctors say, "I let the patient decide among the options"— something that should be self-evident — what they are really saying is, "I avoid giving my patients my definitive opinion." You need information from your doctor and you are paying for an opinion. The way to tell the difference between a doctor who is involving you in the decision-making process and one who is asking too much of you is to look for a clear suggestion by the doctor of a best course of action, at least two or more equivalent options, or options with varying trade-offs of benefits and risks that the doctor clearly explains. All that said, no doctor should do something that he or she does not believe in just because you want it. Though it's rare, some doctors are overly compliant and that's just as problematic as those who are too dogmatic. Every therapeutic option has nuances, and your doctor should be prepared to explain them in a way that helps you make the best decision for your life.

If a doctor is not providing a definitive opinion, it is possible that he or she is not totally comfortable treating the problem you have, fears being blamed for a bad outcome, or is anxious about something else altogether. The reason the doctor avoids offering his or her best opinion matters less than the outcome: Again, it is an opinion that you are paying for, and your doctor's opinion is critical to your ability to make the best choices possible. And that might mean the difference between life and death.

Keep in mind that opinions are shaped not only by facts and knowledge, but also by current and past life experiences. An 80-year-old patient may have a very different outlook on life than his or her 40-year-old (or possibly younger) doctor. *Quality* of life may be more important to the older patient, while *quantity* of life may be more important to the younger patient with school-age children at home, or vice versa.

Similarly, try as they might to remain objective, doctors have emotional responses. For example, a doctor might shy away from a more aggressive therapy after having had a recent bad experience with another patient.

Your part is to tell your doctor what is important to *you*. Saying, "Look, I have lived a nice long life. What I am really concerned about is making sure that my family does not see me in pain," is very different from saying, "I want to fight this cancer with every ounce of my being, and I want a total cure."

The same doctor might give very different opinions depending on the patient's expressed priorities. But make no mistake; *the doctor should give his or her definitive opinion about the best course of action in your case.* You don't necessarily have to base your decisions on your doctor's opinion, but it's important that you know what that opinion is, and what it was based on. And if you choose not to follow your doctor's advice, it's even more important to understand why you're making that decision.

Bringing it all together

Taking charge of your healthcare means thinking about how your loved ones, your doctors, their staff, and your insurance company can best work to improve your health. Each of these groups will likely respond positively to your leadership. Finding the best doctor for you is incredibly important, but it takes some work. Make sure you are treated with respect, communication is clear, and people follow through. Understand what you need, but also what your doctor needs in order to best help you. Define who your main cancer doctor will be, and which doctor will be the point person for any other problems that arise.

NOTES

NOTES

40

CHAPTER 3

What Your Doctor Wants to Know

When going to see your doctor, it always helps to know what information he or she will need. In this chapter, I illustrate the format that doctors use to organize and document the information that you provide. This should help you to better prepare for a more efficient and effective visit. First, know your body. Many of us don't pay much attention to our body. In order to prepare for any medical visit you must be able to quickly and accurately describe physical and mental issues. Otherwise, how can the doctor help you?

Second, prepare for an interactive session. Bring information and plan to ask questions, as well as answer the doctor's questions. This chapter is about the information you need to bring and what types of questions the doctor might ask. During medical visits all parties have to actively participate; and through proper preparation there can be great synergy among the participants.

Let's focus on how to prepare the information that you need to convey to the doctor. In practice, this is actually a straightforward task. Just ask yourself why you are going to see the doctor, then put the relevant information into a clear, succinct story. It would be helpful to write the information down in order to organize your thoughts and ensure that your story is complete once you get into the doctor's office. This can be in outline form or prose. Make sure your story is cohesive and generally in chronological order.

Think about it it: Why might you lose interest in a book or movie? Generally, it's either because you have to work hard to understand the sequence of events, the characters are not developed, or the storyline is so disorganized that you can't make any sense of why or when the storyteller has chosen to tell you a particular piece of information. Your doctor is human, and the same applies to the story you tell during your visit; it can either be relevant, complete, and compelling or disorganized, incomplete and inaccurate.

You are the one in control of the story; doctors can only facilitate and interpret the information. Therefore, be as specific as possible. Avoid saying things like, "Oh, I guess my stomach has been hurting for quite a while." This doesn't define a specific time-frame and, therefore, doesn't have a specific medical meaning. It is better to say: "The pain started 2 months ago" or give your best estimate: "I'm not sure, but I think I had one day of pain about 3 months ago, then about 6 weeks ago it returned and has been present ever since." This will help your doctor gather information in a relatively structured format.

Format of a Doctor's Note

Chief Complaint (CC)

Exactly what problem or issue prompted you to come into the doctor's office at this particular time, and why?

This should be a succinct statement of the reason you have come to see this particular doctor at this particular time. Think back to Claire, who we met at the beginning of the book. She might have told her gastroenterologist: "My family doctor (doctor's name) sent me to have my first screening colonoscopy." A great deal of information is packed into that one sentence. The gastroenterologist now knows (1) who referred her and to whom to communicate the results, (2) that Claire is probably 50 years old, a typical time to begin initial screening, and (3) she likely does not have symptoms or signs of her potential problem (colon cancer).

History of Present Illness (HPI)

The full story of your current problem

For this section and the Past Medical/Surgical History section that follows, request that copies of your medical records, including test results, office notes, and CD-ROM copies or actual films of imaging tests such as **CAT scans** or **MRIs** be sent directly to *you* before the visit. Having results sent directly to you is often better than having them sent to your doctor's office, as long as you do it well before your visit. Like socks in a dryer, medical records can disappear if they are sent directly to a doctor's office. Losing medical records is less likely to occur if you are able to keep track of them. Not only can you keep a copy of your own records, allowing you to easily provide them to all your doctors, you can send or, if you have time, hand-deliver a copy to the doctor's office before your visit. Then you can be sure the records got there and that the doctor had time to review them. Also, bring extra copies with you the day of your visit. However, if for some reason it is not possible to have them sent to you, have them sent to the doctor's office and follow up with a phone call before your visit to make sure they got there.

When your doctor prompts you to provide the HPI (though they may not use this term), begin with either relevant past medical issues, such as, "I was born with ulcerative colitis" (a condition that predisposes to colon cancer) or describe the first manifestation of the problem at hand. The HPI that Claire will tell the surgeon she sees after the gastroenterologist visit might be: "I was feeling fine, without any problems, and was referred to 'Dr. Gastroenterologist,' who performed a routine screening colonoscopy. He found three polyps and one came back as cancer."

Pertinent history, such as the fact that she was feeling fine, is important. A different patient might respond: "For about the past two months, I had maroon-colored stool and weakness. My wife said that I looked pale and I wasn't sure what was wrong. So last month I went to my primary care physician. She said I was anemic (had a low hemoglobin and red blood cell count) and sent me to have a colonoscopy by "Dr. Gastroenterologist," who found the cancer in my colon." The doctor will then guide you to answer other questions about possible related symptoms.

This will go back and forth, and your job will be to succinctly describe the following aspects of your symptoms and signs:

Location	Where in your body did the symptom or sign start? Where is it now?
Radiation	Does the sensation (pain, etc.) move or radiate to another part of your body?
Timing	When did it start? Did it end and, if so, when?
Frequency	How often has it occurred? Is it intermittent or constant? Is it predictable?
Modifiability	Does anything make it better or worse?
Prior Assessment	Have you seen a physician previously for it? If so, have you received a diagnosis? Have you taken any medication or other treatments? If so, what has been the effect?

Past Medical/Surgical History (PMH/PSH)

What medical or surgical problems do you or have you had?

Again, be as specific and complete as you can. For example, write:

- *Pneumonia, age 41*
- *High blood pressure, diagnosed age 44, well-controlled with medication*
- *Diabetes, diagnosed age 47, difficult to control, blood sugars usually 200 to 250, last hemoglobin A1C checked 2 months ago was 8.6*

Family History

What medical problems run in your family?

Depending on your age, you should try to provide information at least two generations above and below you (your grandparents, parents, children and grandchildren) as well as blood-related aunts, uncles and cousins. Make it more extensive if you think it is relevant. List all major problems, but most important are those relevant to your current condition. For example, write:

- *Maternal grandmother, adult-onset diabetes in her 50s, died of stroke age 80*
- *Father, hypertension age 48, heart attack age 60, died of lung cancer age 69*

Medications

What medications do you take?

List current and important past medications, dosages, and how often you take them. Bring medication bottles to your visit. Also include supplements and any over-the-counter (OTC) medications. For example, you might write:

–*Metoprolol 50mg by mouth twice per day*
–*Metformin 1000mg by mouth twice per day*

Allergies

Do any medications or other substances cause a reaction, and what happens during the reaction?

For example, you might write:

–*Sulfa-containing antibiotics caused a red itchy rash all over my body for about three days; this happened when I was 9 years old and I haven't taken any since.*

The above sections represent much of the information you will be asked to provide. Your doctor will either ask you for other relevant information or will obtain it by examining you or ordering medical tests. Obviously, a patient with a long history of cancer or any other chronic illness can have a complex story to tell. Just remember to keep it as simple, specific, and yet complete as possible.

Try to tell your story and ask questions as the doctor is sitting and relaxed. Often patients discuss very important topics after the doctor has stood up and is just about to leave the room. Like a bad dance partner, sometimes the doctor does not make the tempo of the visit very clear and ends the visit abruptly. Other times the patient is embarrassed or fearful about bringing the particular subject to the doctor's attention. However, sometimes it's unavoidable, such as if the patient thinks of the issue at the end of the visit. The pre-visit preparation strategies should help minimize "last minute" comments and questions.

Information About Medications

Another area of common confusion is medications. You should be familiar with key facts about medications. Ideally you should bring all of your medications, including over-the-counter (OTC) medications and supplements to each doctor's visit. If it is impractical to bring your actual medications or you prefer to simply bring a list, please make sure your list is complete and includes medication name, dosage, route of administration (orally, for example) and how often it is taken.

Anatomy of a Prescription

What all those abbreviations mean

In addition to your name, date of birth, gender, the doctor's name, address, phone number, and typically NPI and/or DEA numbers, here is what information a prescription contains that tells the pharmacist what you need. Many of the letters are Latin abbreviations. In the example below, Sig. stands for *signa* (write on label), route of administration, p.o. stands for *per os* (orally), and frequency of administration, q.d. stands for for *quaque die* (every day). There might be specific areas on the prescription for some of the information below and not necessarily four lines, but basically it should look something like this:

Line 1 Medication name, formulation, and strength

Line 2 How the medication should be taken

Line 3 The quantity of medication to be dispensed

Line 4 The number of refills approved

For example, if a doctor wants a patient to take one baby aspirin by mouth once per day and writes for a 30-day supply with one refill, though there might be minor stylistic differences, the prescription will read:

Line 1	ASA 81 mg tabs
Line 2	Sig. Ŧ p.o. q.d.
Line 3	Disp #30
Line 4	Refill x 1

Usually a doctor writes a prescription for medications that must be dispensed by a pharmacist; however, sometimes a doctor writes a prescription for OTC medications or supplements. Medications usually have a trade name (what the pharmaceutical or biotechnology company sells it as) and a generic name (what the molecule is called).

If a medication patent expires, other companies can then make a generic version of the original medication. In this situation, the original pharmaceutical company might sell it by its trade name (possibly at a premium price) and other companies might sell the active molecule compounded with other agents as a generic, typically with its own trade name as well. Companies that make generic drugs must prove bio-equivalence, meaning that equivalent doses of the generic formulation should lead to equivalent levels of the active molecule in the patient's body compared to the original formulation. For many medications the generic and original brand name versions are interchangeable. However, for some medications, the brand name and generic versions act differently in the body. Some doctors are more attuned to this than others. You should discuss this with your physician.

Biologically-engineered therapies (sometimes called **biological therapies** or **targeted therapies**) are typically produced by living cells. There are no "generic" versions, but when the patent expires on these medications there can be "biosimilar" versions. The **Food and Drug Administration** (FDA) is currently working with phamaceutical and biotechnology companies to define the particular requirements that a biological therapy must meet to be called "biosimilar". I again discuss generics and biosimilars in *Chapter 5—Making Treatment Decisions.*

For many medications you can ask for samples. As you may know, pharmaceutical representatives sometimes leave medication samples in doctors' offices to be dispensed directly to patients. Often these medications can help with various issues: (1) To determine whether you can tolerate the medication before you fill the prescription; (2) If you have a mail order pharmacy plan, this can allow you to start taking the medication while you are waiting for the medication to be delivered; (3) Samples can supplement a patient's supply of medication. Beware: medication samples are usually not monitored by a pharmacist. Please make sure that you are getting the correct medication, the correct dose, and that the expiration date has not passed.

NOTES

54

CHAPTER 4

Understanding Your Medical Condition

ASKING THE RIGHT QUESTIONS

Let's go back to Claire for a moment. When we last saw her, her doctor had just told her that she has cancer. By the time she arrives at home the first shock has begun to fade, and she's starting to think of all sorts of questions she wishes she had asked. She goes online and starts surfing the Internet, looking for information about colon cancer. She finds some answers, which raise even more questions.

Claire's response to her diagnosis is not unusual. Many recently diagnosed patients—and just as many people who only suspect they have cancer—turn to the Internet. It's fast. It's easy. Sometimes it's even accurate. Some patients find it helpful and comforting to go online before knowing all the facts. Reading up about the disease they have—or might have— gives them a sense of control, the feeling that they're doing something positive. And in many cases online research can be helpful, particularly in helping the patient frame the questions to ask the doctor. However, many find searching for answers when they aren't even certain what kind of cancer they have emotionally draining, and reading specific details about the disease or its treatment—which may or may not pertain to them—can be counterproductive.

There are a multitude of cancer types, subtypes, locations, stages, and potential treatments. Searching for information before you know the facts of your particular situation can provoke unrealistic fears—or equally false optimism. Neither are helpful. Asking questions is good and important. Asking the *right* questions of the person who knows your particular situation best—your doctor—is critical to being an informed and engaged patient. Though you will probably have many more questions, I have included some key ones below that you should ask.

What is my diagnosis and what type of tumor do I have?

The first thing you need to know is whether or not you have cancer, one of the various conditions that may lead to it, a benign tumor, or no cancer at all. If you are not sure, ask your doctor. If you have cancer, ask for your specific diagnosis.

Knowing your diagnosis means knowing exactly what type of tumor or cancer you have. Not all tumors are cancer, and not all cancers have **solid tumors** associated with them. For example, leukemia is a **liquid tumor**. Many separate cancer cells float throughout your body in your bone marrow and bloodstream.

All cancers start in a particular organ or type of tissue such as lung, liver, colon, etc. When someone asks what kind of cancer you have, what he or she is asking is: "Where did your cancer start?" Occasionally, particularly in the case of fast-growing, aggressive cancers, it is impossible to tell in which tissue your cancer originated. If you don't already know, ask your doctor which specific type of cancer you have and write it down. Then ask if there are any subtypes of your tumor, and if so, which one you have. Ask for a copy of your **pathology report**, and ask your doctor to go over it with you.

What stage is my cancer?

Understanding your **cancer stage** is key to understanding your treatment plan. For example, if you have a small cancer confined to your breast, surgery alone might be enough. The problem is that no one can say for sure whether the cancer *is* confined. When it comes to tumors, size usually *does* matter; typically the larger the tumor, the more likely it is to have metastasized. However, sometimes small tumors have already metastasized, whereas large ones might not have. That's why for most cancers staging is important.

The process of determining stage varies with the type of cancer. For many cancers "staging" the cancer means getting imaging studies such as a **CAT scan** or **MRI** to detect where in your body metastases might be hiding. Not all cancer types require this kind of testing, and there are different staging systems for different cancers, but the most commonly used system for solid tumors is Tumor-Node-Metastasis (TNM).

TUMOR: Your doctor will determine the size of your tumor, and whether or not there has been direct growth past the outer edge of that organ into the immediate surrounding area, to help determine your cancer stage.

NODE: The doctor will then try to determine whether the cancer has spread to **lymph nodes**.

METASTASIS: Finally, your doctor will try to determine whether your cancer has spread to organs other than the one where your cancer began.

Because cancers can vary enormously in terms of aggressiveness, the implications of the stage of each type of cancer also varies enormously. One example not necessarily associated with any tumor type, T1N1M0 (pronounced T one, N one, M zero), translates to something like: "The tumor is less than 'X' centimeters in diameter; it has spread to the lymph node chain closest to the original tumor; and there are no distant metastases." For this particular tumor type, based on the TNM staging, this patient has stage II cancer. Again, this is just an example of the nomenclature, it's not meant to suggest that T1N1M0 defines a stage II tumor. Depending on the tumor type, various tumors might have different TNM scores and still be stage II.

Most cancers have four potential stages, typically written I, II, III and IV. Stage I is the earliest and typically has a much better **prognosis**. Stage IV is the latest, and typically means the tumor has already metastasized. Some cancers will need to be "re-staged" after treatment. Again, all of these concepts are discussion points for you to have with your doctor.

The doctor can usually say that a particular stage of a particular tumor type is *statistically* associated with a certain rate of survival. This means that "Y" percent of all patients with stage II disease are alive, let's say, five years after diagnosis. This percentage could be close to 100 percent or dramatically lower, depending on the particular tumor type.

For some types of tumors this percentage can be quite accurate; for others there could be a large degree of variability. In addition, it is important to remember that this calculation is based on statistics from a *group* of patients, and it might not apply to you in particular.

Knowing your cancer's stage can help determine appropriate treatment. In our example, doctors might treat stage II disease with therapies A, B, and C. They might choose different therapies for stages I, III, or IV. Staging systems are not static; as we learn more about cancer staging systems are often revised and improved. You should ask your doctor to explain the stage of your cancer and what information that provides.

What is the natural history of my cancer?

You might ask: "So what would happen to me if I did not take any of the treatments offered?" The answer probably is that the cancer would grow and spread, and your condition would continue to worsen. Almost everyone with cancer should get treatment quickly, but for a few types of indolent (slow-growing) cancers, watchful waiting (continuing to monitor without specific treatment) is appropriate. For some types of cancers, watchful waiting is appropriate when the tumor is in a slow growth phase, but treatment should occur when or if a rapid growth phase begins. It's helpful to understand how the particular cancer that you have is likely to affect you now and over time, based on what is known about how it affects people in general.

Sometimes other tests can be used in addition to staging to better determine your prognosis. These are typically recently developed tests aimed at determining whether your tumor contains certain mutated genes. The results might affect your prognosis, depending on the gene and whether a mutation is found. Certain gene mutations help to guide the physician and patient to more effective therapies. Indeed, we are on our way to fulfilling the promise of **personalized medicine** (discussed further in *Chapter 10: Looking Forward*).

It is important to understand how fast your tumor is likely to grow. Some tumors grow over years; others over months; and some aggressive cancers grow over weeks. Tumor growth can be irregular. The growth of some cancers proceeds to a point and then plateaus. Also, you will want to know about the pattern of spread (whether and to which organs your cancer might metastasize). Finally, you might ask whether the growth of your cancer is likely to accelerate with time. Some patients diagnosed with incurable cancer want to know what exactly will happen to their body as their tumor grows and spreads. They may want to know if the type of tumor they have can cause death, and if so, how exactly the tumor does this. Try to determine what level of knowledge will be most helpful to you, and guide your doctor on this topic.

What is my prognosis?

As with any question in this book, but especially with this one, you need to ask yourself why you are asking for this information, and determine whether and how it might help you. As mentioned earlier, this book is meant to guide you to the best questions *for you*. For most people it is helpful at some point to know their prognosis—that is, how healthy they can expect to be and for how long, as well as how long they have to live. The challenge is that doctors can only give you an answer based on statistics (what studies tell them about how groups of people who have the type and stage of cancer you have fare in general).

Your prognosis is unlikely to be exactly accurate because it is based on others' experiences, and may not account for the factors unique to your situation. Patients inherently sense this fact. Because a prognosis is an informed "best guess" estimate that often doesn't account for the unique features of your experience, information about your prognosis isn't always pro- ductive. For example, knowing your prognosis might reinforce an overly optimistic or pessimistic outlook.

This can happen when the doctor *miscommuni- cates* information. Some doctors don't like giving bad news, so they either avoid it or provide a more opti- mistic scenario. In other cases, the doctor may feel that under promising by offering a pessimistic prognosis and then over delivering with a better-than-expected outcome is the best policy. Finally, some doctors simply do not relay information clearly, and they do not check to see if their patients understood what was conveyed.

Prognoses can also be potentially harmful when the patient *misunderstands* information. Most people really want everything to be okay. Mishearing information is not uncommon. The brain sometimes subconsciously permits a patient or family member to selectively hear only certain information or process information in an irrational way. Biology plays a role in this. Patients with cancer are often stressed. This triggers the release of adrenaline, which can cause hyperawareness and potentially a "fight-or-flight" response.

While this can be helpful in some situations, very high levels of adrenaline can harm a patient's ability to process the full spectrum of information about the current situation. At its best, the hyperawareness associated with a surge of adrenaline can help you "live in the moment," focusing on what will improve the odds of survival *in that moment*. This can help you to focus, which is good. However, it can also cause you to consider all threats imminent. The ensuing response might be to prepare for battle (fight) or to take off in the other direction (flight).

This panicked response can be mental

or physical. Stressed patients may literally be unable to hear or process bad news, no matter how skillfully the doctor presents it. On the other hand, the patient might be devastated by news that is not really that bad. When this happens, the patient may have a completely inaccurate recollection of what was said during the appointment.

Recognizing adrenaline's role in your body and managing its potentially negative effects, while leveraging its positive effects, is critical. This can be as simple as reminding yourself to stay calm or discussing the situation with your care partner. The more you can stay in control during the visit, the more effectively you can understand your doctor—and make sure your doctor understands you. Also, your care partner can be invaluable as a second pair of ears to hear and process the information being communicated during the visit.

Let's assume for a minute that both you and your doctor are dealing effectively with reality. If the doctor informs you that of all people with your type and stage of cancer, 80 percent—or eight out of every ten patients—are alive ten years after diagnosis, your next logical question might be: "What's the difference between the eight who are alive after ten years and the two who aren't, and where does my condition fit into that scenario?" Knowing this might give you a better sense of your particular chances of surviving past year ten. Remember, that's what it will be: a chance.

However, what if 50 percent, or five out of every ten people with your type and stage of cancer, are alive five years after diagnosis? A prognosis like this can be hard to process, particularly if there are no identifiable factors that separate the 50 percent who are alive five years later from the 50 percent who are not. Still, having this information might help you in fighting your cancer more effectively, in planning out life in general, and as motivation for getting the most out of life, however long it lasts.

Let's consider another scenario. A 90-year-old woman visits her doctor and is informed that there is an abnormality in her blood and it might be cancer. The doctor wants to do more testing. He says that if he finds cancer, there is a 50 percent chance that it will take her life in five years. There is a cure, but the therapy has an upfront mortality risk of 5 percent, or one in every 20 people will die within one month of receiving the therapy. This patient might say that she loves life, her affairs are in order, and the bad news of a confirmed diagnosis of cancer and potentially harsh therapies might be worse for her than the potential benefit of treatment. If this woman cannot use the news about her diagnosis and prognosis to live a better life, she might not want to know, and that might be the best approach *in this particular case.*

In other instances, doctors and patients might not focus on the right disease. For example, if a 60-year-old patient has a cancer with a 60 percent five-year mortality rate—meaning that after five years, only four out of ten patients will be alive—that would not be good news. But if that same patient has had three heart attacks and severe heart failure, he might have a 90 percent five-year mortality from the heart disease—meaning that after five years only one out of ten patients will be alive—based on his heart condition alone. In other words, he is more likely to die from his heart condition than from his cancer. The risk of dying is so often associated with cancer that sometimes patients and doctors underestimate the risk of dying from other diseases. Appreciating this can be important in making sure the correct expectations and appropriate level of treatment is provided for each disease.

Can anything improve my prognosis?

My patients often ask if choosing one treatment or therapy over another can alter their prognosis. The answer is 'yes,' your prognosis might change over time for various reasons. Doctors often use five years from the time of diagnosis as a milestone. If additional information about your type of cancer comes to light in those years, your prognosis might change.

Your body's response to treatment might also alter your prognosis; patients who are cancer-free at that important five-year milestone are often considered cured. This may or may not be true; certainly it is not possible to know with 100 percent accuracy in any case, but passing the five-year milestone cancer-free is always a great sign. If you have questions about your prognosis, or think it might have changed, ask your doctor about it. *Chapter 5: Making Treatment Decisions* deals extensively with making treatment decisions with your doctor.

How long do I have to live?

This is one of the first questions many patients ask. Many doctors respond that this cannot be known for sure, but patients in a similar situation typically have "X" long to live. Death can be one of the most difficult things to discuss, particularly with a doctor you have just met. However, in some ways the first visit with your doctor can be a good time to discuss this subject. Early in this new relationship your doctor and you might find it easier to be objective about your long-term outlook, since there might not a strong emotional connection between the two of you yet.

Can my cancer be cured?

You might also ask whether your cancer can be cured, and what the chances of that would be.

Would you please review my scans and other test results with me?

A picture is worth a lot of words—just look at the report your radiologist dictates based on your MRI scan. Looking at the actual MRIs, CAT scans, or other types of imaging of your body can help you understand where the cancer is located and why certain therapies are needed or perhaps cannot be done. For example, if a tumor is very close to a major blood vessel surgery might not be the best option, as it would risk injury to the blood vessel. Ask your doctor to view your scans and review the results of other diagnostic tests with you.

When a tumor is removed, the surgeon sends it to a pathologist who cuts it into paper-thin slices, stains them, and looks at them under a microscope. It's probably not practical or informative to see pathology slides of the tumor that has been removed, but having your doctor walk you through the pathologists's written report can be very enlightening.

How are my symptoms related to my disease?

A man with pancreatic cancer walks into the doctor's office because his skin and the whites of his eyes have turned yellow, and he is experiencing grayish diarrhea that floats. What's wrong? The doctor will first determine which organs and anatomical structures have compromised function. In this case, a tumor is in the pancreas near the stomach and small intestine, and it is pushing on the bile duct, which takes bile from the liver and gallbladder to the intestine to help with digestion.

A blocked bile duct cannot deliver bile to the intestine, and bile literally backs up into the liver and bloodstream, causing the person to become yellow (jaundiced) from the color of the bile. Furthermore, if bile and pancreatic juices are not able to get to the intestine, then the patient is not able to absorb many of the nutrients in the food that he is eating—which can cause diarrhea.

The patient should next ask the doctor about possible symptom remedies, such as surgery, medication, etc. For example, taking digestive enzymes by mouth may help the patient feel better and absorb more nutrients. Allowing the bile to flow freely may require placing a stent (a tube to bypass the blockage) or removing the tumor. You might also ask whether

these symptoms and **signs** must be treated. See also:
Chapter 5: Making Treatment Decisions.

Who will be the main doctor in charge of my care?

As discussed previously, it is important to determine the answer to this question early. For the most part, one doctor is in charge for each medical problem or course of treatment. However, in some instances this issue can be complex, and occasionally it is necessary to have two or more doctors working closely together on a specific issue. For example, the main doctor who keeps track of whether and when a **screening test** such as a colonoscopy is needed might be the primary care physician (PCP), typically an internist or family practice physician. The PCP may refer the patient to a gastroenterologist, who will be the point person for the colonoscopy and interpreting the results.

If the gastroenterologist diagnoses colon cancer, the PCP or the gastroenterologist might refer the patient to a medical oncologist, who will likely help find a surgical oncologist, oversee the chemotherapy if needed, and be in charge of overall cancer care. This scenario is typical, but there are local practice variations regarding who takes charge and at what stage. While it is usually not helpful to be dogmatic about the issue, establishing each team member's role is crucial. To refer back to our corporate analogy, in most businesses an employee reports to a specific person in charge, but sometimes there are "dotted lines" that connect peers or employees in different divisions and offices. It might even be helpful to draw an organizational chart as you would see in a company, to visually demonstrate the relationships among the team members.

What contributed to or caused my cancer?

As we discussed at the beginning of this book, many chemicals and environmental factors can contribute to or cause cancer. If smoking contributed, you can stop. If a chemical exposure at work contributed, you can avoid it. If genetics had something to do with it, others in your family might need to be screened for the presence of a tumor, or genetic mutation that predisposes them to cancer. Many times, however, there is no identifiable contributing factor. Some people feel guilty about specific behaviors that might have contributed to their cancer. This feeling is common but usually not particularly productive. Maybe your actions contributed to your cancer; maybe they didn't. Try not to get caught up in blaming yourself. It's more helpful to think: "Okay, I can't change the past. So where do we go from here to try to make my future better?"

Are my children or other relatives at increased risk of developing cancer?

Many times the answer is either that there is a small increased risk and no one knows how to modify it, or there is no known increased risk to your children or other family members. Of course, sometimes there is a predictable increased risk depending on whether you harbor a genetic mutation in your DNA, and in some cases your children can be tested for the genetic mutation. Lots of thought should go into this decision.

For example, if your children test positive (have the genetic mutation that increases their risk of developing cancer), is there anything that can be done to alter the risk? Will a positive test result affect their eligibility to purchase insurance? How will they feel for the rest of their life? **Genetic counselors**, though they may not be doctors, typically have advanced training in helping patients and families understand genetic testing. A genetic counselor can help you sort through whether testing would be helpful, and can then help interpret the results if you decide to have the testing done.

Should I get a second opinion?

You might not need to ask this question, but it is good to consider how you feel about the issue. Do you feel you need a second opinion from another doctor? Many patients trust their doctor completely and do not question his or her judgment. However, it is healthy and important to question your doctor's thinking and explore his or her reasoning. In some cases, doctors encourage patients to question them not because they aren't confident, but because they want to make sure their patients are comfortable with and believe in the treatment plan. I don't mind when patients ask whether they should get a second opinion. If they are asking me this question, it means they *really* trust me. The vast majority of patients never ask this question, and in most cases it is not relevant; the patient is getting great care and there is no need for a second opinion.

However, there are times when a patient has a rare manifestation of a rare type of tumor or needs very specific therapy that is not offered at the institution where he or she is receiving treatment. In these cases, the patient and even the doctor might want a second opinion. The doctor might call a colleague, or present the patient's case at a weekly conference at his or her own institution, but occasionally it may be in the patient's best interest to get part or all of the treatment elsewhere. No doctor or institution is the best choice for every situation, though most major medical centers and teaching hospitals can handle almost all of the cases that walk through the door.

Many brilliant doctors in private practice, particularly those not affiliated with academic institutions, do not have as much experience with rare diseases as doctors at major teaching or research hospitals, where patients with rare diseases are often referred for more specialized care. In some cases, the private practice doctor refers the patient to a sub-specialist at a teaching hospital. Usually the private practice doctor, the doctor at the teaching hospital, and the patient decide together how best to proceed. Many times both doctors follow along together. Alternatively the academic doctor may see the patient once, and from then on care is administered by the private practitioner, unless care is best administered entirely at the academic teaching center. Many factors go into this decision, such as how far the patient lives from each doctor, and whether the patient will enroll in a clinical trial, which is usually administered at the academic medical center (though sometimes these are done in a private doctor's office). The bottom line is that the arrangement needs to be one that best serves the patient's needs.

What can I do to improve my chances of living a longer, healthier life?

Patients want to know what they can do to improve their chances of living longer, healthier lives. First, learn strategies to reduce and manage the anxiety that dealing with cancer can cause. Second, be inquisitive and critical in your approach to understanding your current situation and making medical decisions. Develop a sense of what to take at face value and what not to; that's what this book is about. Third, determine whether you are engaged in any activity or are exposed to anything that is harming your health. If so, work to modify or reduce that exposure. Fourth, focus on appropriate dietary intake and exercise. Though you may not always be able to quantify the effects of living a healthier lifestyle, you will probably feel the positive physical and psychological results, and every little bit does help.

Maybe you've heard somebody say, "I already have lung cancer, so why should I quit smoking now?" The answer is simple: Most therapies have some sort of potential toxicity. These toxicities may be quite significant and even life-threatening. Hence, it is important to maximize your ability to tolerate a potentially toxic therapy that may offer substantial benefit. For this reason, now is the time to get in the best shape that you can. A patient with lung cancer may not be able to get the operation he needs because he continues to smoke and has poor lung function. Improving your overall health may be a key contribution that you can make toward treating your cancer, and it will likely give you peace of mind knowing that you are doing your part to save your own life.

NOTES

76

Making Treatment Decisions and Building Your Action Plan

What are my treatment goals?

The goal of any therapy is to accomplish one or more of these three things: (1) to try to cure you, (2) to help you live longer, (3) to help you feel better. It is crucial to establish your goals *clearly* with your doctor, and ask about the likelihood of success if you take the proposed treatment. By taking the proposed therapy you might be aiming for a cure, a **partial response,** a **complete response**, or simply to stabilize the tumor size. Alternatively, you might expect to simply feel more energy or breathe easier.

Once you establish treatment goals, you can figure out which questions to ask to determine how each treatment will affect your overall course. Though goals should be rational, realistic, and attainable, the pace of discovery of cancer treatments is accelerating dramatically, and treatments that we couldn't have dreamed of just a few years ago are breakthrough treatments today. It is very likely that new treatments will be available during the time you are living with cancer; therefore, your goals might change over time. The idea is to understand your particular medical condition and what treatment options are available, then make the best decision you can. In a 50-year-old with colon cancer that has spread to the liver and lung, for example, living to be 90 is probably not a realistic goal…yet.

However, it might be entirely possible to shrink the tumors enough with chemotherapy so that surgery could remove them and chemotherapy could be stopped for a period of time. That approach might help the patient live long enough to enter a clinical trial of an as-yet-unreleased treatment, which could help make bigger strides against the cancer. Every response to treatment, every victory, no matter how small, can be very important. Ask your doctor to help you set your therapeutic goals as early as possible.

What are my treatment options?

When setting your initial treatment goals, it is important to consider what type of cancer you have, your prognosis, and which therapies are available. You and your doctor will want to discuss a fairly comprehensive list of the available treatment options, and consider each one carefully to determine which ones will give you the best shot at achieving your treatment goals. However, for some cancers at certain stages there are well-researched therapies that are the "standard of care," meaning that one particular treatment regimen is offered to most people in your position and there will not be many options to choose among. The focus here should be for you to feel comfortable that you have the whole story.

If your doctor informs you that the suggested therapy for your cancer results in a 95 percent cure rate, and this has been established through research done over the last 25 years, this is good, and it probably does not makes sense to stress too much or exhaust yourself researching other treatment options for hours.

However, there are many situations where potential therapies span the spectrum in terms of effectiveness and potential **adverse reactions** (also known as **side effects**). In these situations, it is crucial for you to be confident that your doctor is well-read on the nuances of one therapy compared to the others available. For all therapies, only some patients will respond. For example, of all patients with a particular type of cancer, those without a particular mutation in their DNA might respond to one medication, while those that have that particular mutation might respond better to a different therapy available only through a clinical trial. If this situation applies to you, it is really important that both you and your doctor understand where you fall on this spectrum, and which therapy applies and why. Finally, in some situations, it is the potential side effects of the medications that dictate the best therapy, and not the effectiveness of one therapy compared to another.

What are the benefits and risks of each treatment?

In considering various treatment options, a major question is: What are the chances that this particular treatment will achieve its intended goal, and what are the potential adverse events and their chances of occurring? For example, if you have esophageal cancer that is interfering with swallowing and the treatment goal is to allow you to eat, then placing a stent into the esophagus to bypass the tumor might help.

The success rate (chance of being able to swallow) might be "X" percent. The complication rate (risk of an adverse event such as inadvertently perforating the esophagus during the placement of a stent) might be "Y" percent. Finally, the mortality rate or risk of dying from the procedure might be "Z" percent.

Determining how to weigh the benefits versus the risks might take some work. In addition, sometimes the risks are not known for a given therapy, procedure, or combination of therapies, particularly those that are experimental.

The example above regarding esophageal stent placement is relatively straightforward. However, you can imagine how decisions can be difficult for the doctor, not to mention the patient, when multiple combinations of treatments are available, each with its own chance of "success" and various potential adverse events to consider.

It is important to go into detail about these issues with your doctor. It is critical that you clearly understand all risks and benefits by the end of the visit, because after the visit the doctor is no longer present to clarify things. Of course you can always call or schedule another visit to ask further questions, but the more answers you can get per visit, the more confident you are going to feel as you make decisions when you talk things over with your family.

Since combination chemotherapy regimens can require multiple medications to be given together, when considering these regimens, you should find out what "success" means for the regimen as a whole—but you should also find out the potential adverse events for each individual medication in that regimen.

Can I tolerate treatment?

Most cancer patients just want the cancer out of their bodies and will do anything to make that happen. But a major question to ask is whether that is possible and, if so, if your body and mind can tolerate the therapies you need in order to accomplish that goal. One major question that many patients, and occasionally doctors, forget to consider is what *other* medical problems the patient has that might affect his or her ability to survive the therapy and avoid becoming dramatically debilitated. The first step is to consider all current and past medical problems and medications, and make a judgment about the impact of these on treatment of the cancer, as well as the impact of cancer treatment on these other medical problems or medications. Your doctor is the best person to consult about how to keep you as safe as possible during therapy. Modifying risk factors where possible can improve certain performance criteria, such as endurance, in order to get ready for the treatment. Alternatively, a patient might choose to go ahead with therapy despite significant risks posed by other medical problems that cannot be improved prior to therapy. Asking questions will lead to an informed decision.

What is the treatment timeline?

The timing of therapy always matters, and sometimes it matters more than others. Radiation or chemotherapy is often given in multiple doses over time using a specific schedule that has been researched to make the treatment more effective or safer.

Adjuvant therapy is given *after* another therapy. For example, adjuvant chemotherapy may be given after surgery to attempt to eradicate errant cancer cells that could not be seen and, therefore, were not removed at the time of the operation. In this case, the tumor cells might have extended just past the margin where the surgeon cut. Though they might not be visible to the naked eye, they are floating in the blood and bone marrow, or may have formed **micrometastases** in another organ. In contrast, **neoadjuvant** therapy is given *before* another therapy. For example, neoadjuvant chemotherapy is sometimes given before surgery in order to shrink the tumor and make it easier to remove.

How will we determine response?

It is extremely important to discuss with your doctor how you both will determine what your response to therapy has been. This is tied directly to treatment goals, and it helps to set expectations. For example, your doctor may be looking for you to feel better or for your tumor to shrink or maybe disappear. It is important to ask your doctor to define treatment success. Will your tumor be examined by imaging techniques such as MRI or CAT scans? If so, should you expect a partial response, such as a reduction in tumor size, or a complete response, where the tumor has completely disappeared? Another important concept is **disease-free survival**. After a complete response to therapy, how likely will it be that a **relapse** (the tumor coming back) will occur? You will also want to determine a "Plan B" in case you do not achieve your goals.

What impact will this treatment have on my family?

It is not uncommon for family members to suffer as much or more than the patient. There are many reasons for this. First, in a way family members have even less control over the situation than the patient. Typically the patient is the one who is ultimately the decision-maker, including which therapies to accept or refuse, when pain needs treatment, or when to try going to work versus staying home. Moreover, both family members and the patient can feel intense emotions and not know what to do with them.

It's worth acknowledging that though the situation might not be good, it can be confronted. The thing to remember is that going through this experience together with your family is usually best for all involved. However, sometimes the patient and family members need more help than they can provide for each other. Support groups are not for everyone but can be incredibly useful; they can include patients, caregivers, or both. In addition, formal psychotherapy and antidepressant medication can be quite useful for some patients and their family members.

Write down what is on your mind and share it with those you trust. Discussing your emotions first, including fear and anger, can help you get to the root cause of stress. Work with your care partner to anticipate the potential stresses that everyone involved might have, including physical, mental, emotional, spiritual, and financial. It's also important to figure out which parts of life the stress might affect, including relationships, professional life, etc.

One of the biggest advantages of working together on this is the chance to develop realistic expectations and learn more about each other than you've ever known. It's a chance to recommit yourselves to each other, to watch courage in action, and to be there for each other when you need help being brave.

The real question is the same as it was before you developed cancer. Can you turn adversity to advantage? And the answer is the same as well: sometimes yes, sometimes no. But trying to accomplish this is the essence of living a robust, fulfilling life—with or without cancer. Sharing this journey with your family can bring you closer together. That said, there are times when each participant in this fight is likely to need a break, and some time alone. Figuring out when these times occur can be tricky, even for the person that needs the time alone. Giving space while at the same time being there can be a real balancing act.

Will my cancer or its therapy affect my sex life?

It depends; many factors come into play. Some cancers directly affect reproductive organs or diminish libido (desire for sex). Some cancers are more debilitating than others. You may feel too tired to have sex, and some people just don't feel sexy when they think of themselves as a patient. However, being a cancer survivor can be sexy in its own way. It's a little like being a war hero—maybe not in that same "blaze of glory" sense, but in the strength that it implies you have.

People with a healthy sex life before cancer will quite likely have a satisfying sex life following therapy, assuming that they feel physically well. Here, too, open dialogue is the key to preempting and mitigating negative effects. If it's too much to have sex at any given time, just wait it out for a little while, and the desire usually returns. If it does not, consider getting checked out to see if you have a hormonal or other type of physical problem. Hypogonadism (low sex hormones), which can have many dramatic negative effects on men and women including low libido and other medical problems, usually needs to be treated. However, hormone replacement therapy may be harmful with cancers where reproductive hormones, such as estrogen or testosterone, cause the tumor grow. Again, this is something to talk to your doctor about.

Your sexual partner may simply have misconceptions about what you want or what you can do. For example, a man with rectal cancer ends up with a permanent colostomy bag. (A colostomy is a procedure that brings the colon to the abdominal wall to collect feces in a bag, see: "Ostomy" in the Glossary). He is able to have an erection after surgery but his wife no longer initiates contact with him. He assumes it's because she is "turned off" by his colostomy bag. However, she is simply afraid that he cannot tolerate sex. Simple communication, as usual, can often restore a healthy physical and emotional relationship.

Will my cancer therapy affect my fertility?

For some cancer survivors, new beginnings

after successful therapy include having children. If you are in your reproductive years, it's important to determine whether the cancer or its therapy will alter your fertility. And even if you don't want to have a child, some people feel a sense of loss when they can no longer bring life into the world. You might want to consider banking (i.e. freezing) sperm or eggs for use after your cancer therapy. Please discuss all this with your doctor.

How does chemotherapy work?

Most traditional **chemotherapy** actually causes DNA breaks. I know I said that DNA damage causes cancer, but chemotherapy drugs are designed to preferentially work on cancer cells. Since cancer cells are different than normal cells, ideally the chemotherapy "selectively" causes DNA breaks in the cancer cells and kills them, while leaving normal cells alone. However, the selectivity is not perfect.

Hence, if you are receiving chemotherapy for lung cancer, normal cells that replenish your blood, the lining of your intestine, and your hair can all be affected. The result may be side effects such as anemia, infection, nausea, diarrhea, and hair loss. And, as you may have guessed, traditional chemotherapy can, in some cases (though this is not common) *cause* cancer. Typically, though, the very small theoretical risk of another cancer is not a reason to avoid a potentially useful therapy for cancer you have now. However, this is an important issue to discuss with your doctor.

How does radiation therapy work?

Similar to traditional chemotherapy, **radiation therapy** damages DNA in cells, causing them to die. Also, as with chemotherapy, radiation treatments can actually put you at risk for other cancers to develop, but fortunately this is not common. In certain situations, radiation can be given by sitting in front of a machine (usually on more than one occasion) that aims radiation beams at your tumor; this is called external beam radiotherapy.

In contrast to traditional chemotherapy, which treats your entire body, with external beam radiation therapy, the radiation oncologist points the beam at a specific part of the body in order to target the cancer and avoid damaging normal tissue; but again, there is no way to perfect this approach. Alternatively, radiation-emitting objects or substances can be implanted or injected into your body. Each type of tumor responds differently to each type of radiation, and some types of tumors do not respond to radiation therapy at all.

How do biological (targeted) therapies work?

Biological therapies are usually injectable substances designed to mimic or target a particular chemical or protein in the body and either promote or inhibit a particular cellular function. In a way, these therapies leverage the body's own system to fight the tumor. The specificity of a clearly defined target in the body is the main functional difference between this and traditional chemotherapy. Even though biological therapies have clearly defined targets within the body, they have potential adverse effects just like other therapies. As always, a good discussion with your doctor can usually get you the facts you need.

Most biologically-engineered targeted therapies are produced by living organisms such as bacteria, and then purified. There are well worked out manufacturing processes, and these medicines do not generally carry a risk of infection from the manufacturing process. However, some medications that are considered biological therapies are purified from other humans. Immunoglobulin therapy represents this type of biological therapy. They are generally very safe, but it is impossible to completely eliminate the risk of passing on an infectious agent from one human to another. This is not generally a reason to avoid this type of therapy, but understanding the risk of any medication represents an important discussion to have with your doctor.

When patents expire for small molecule, chemically-based therapies, other companies are then allowed to make "generics". The companies need to work with the Food and Drug Administration (FDA) to demonstrate bioequivalence to the original medication. This means that the equivalent blood levels of the active ingredient should be achieved with an equivalent dose. However, with biologically-engineered targeted therapies, the manufacturing process is typically complex, and the actual medication is usually a large, complex molecule that is produced by a living organism. Therefore, as patents on these medications expire, companies who want to "copy" these drugs are going to have to work closely with the FDA to produce a "biosimilar" medication. The approval process for biosimilars will likely be more rigorous than for generics, and individualized depending on the particular medication. Many biological therapy patents are about to expire, and this is an active area of collaboration and negotiation between biotechnology companies and the FDA. Though the goal is to produce a medication that works just as well as the original, there are risks that some biosimilars will not work as well; however, because manufacturing technology has advanced, there is also a chance that the biosimilar will work better than the original. The good news is that the cost of biosimilars will be lower than the original medication, thereby increasing access to these vital medications.

How do immune-based cancer therapies work?

These therapies are designed to alert the patient's immune system to the presence of the tumor. They cause the patient's immune system to target and try to kill the tumor cells in much the same way that the immune system rids the body of an infection. These therapies are being improved and applied to more and more tumors.

How do my doctor and I decide when I have had enough treatment?

Too many patients and doctors do not consider the question of when enough is enough. Some cancer survivors think, "I have cancer and I must constantly try to rid my body of the cancer cells." Patients might feel that if they stop therapy, they are letting down their loved ones, or they might feel like it is their moral obligation to have more therapy. In addition, they might subconsciously feel that if they stop therapy, they will have too much time on their hands and will think of their disease or demise constantly.

Similarly, the doctor might feel that he or she is letting down the patient or their loved ones; or worse, that it is his or her job or moral obligation to administer therapy. Moreover, further therapy might be what the doctor would choose if in the patient's place; he or she might believe that to do anything less is not taking care of the patient.

Like other complex decisions with multiple variables, the decision whether to continue therapy should depend on the patient's goals. However, it is not always clear what should be done to accomplish a particular goal. Moreover, during the course of therapy your goals are likely to change and evolve. There are many potential reasons to consider discontinuing therapy at specific times:

1. If therapy is putting you in imminent danger.

2. If therapy is truly not helping.

3. If you are simply worn out and want to focus *less* on your disease and more on important life events.

Sure, sometimes a patient feels a sense of hopelessness, and just needs some encouragement. In some cases, depression can cause a patient to "give up"; when that happens, the depression should be addressed and treated. But at other times a break from exhausting therapy is essential. Fighting cancer can be harder than any job imaginable; it's physically, mentally, and emotionally exhausting. A break might be exactly what the patient needs to regain the strength to continue the fight. If the decision to stop therapy is made for healthy reasons, it should be respected.

When should I think about end-of-life planning?

The answer, of course, is throughout life. Most of us try to live in the moment, but we recognize that death can come at any time. Either through securing life insurance or some other type of planning, we acknowledge and, to a greater or lesser extent, plan for that moment. Of course patients with cancer may have an accelerated timeframe for considering this issue.

For most, it is important to discuss your wishes with those around you, including your doctor and your family. For patients with small children, this issue can pose an incredibly difficult situation. There is a good deal written about helping children deal with the fact that a loved one has cancer and what that might mean, and experts in this area should be consulted. This topic is beyond the scope of this book. Of course, discussions about death can be quite painful, and most people want to keep them to a minimum. But remember, living life is not usually a perfectly even experience. There are poignant and important times in each of our lives, and often we can do an incredible amount of "living" in a very short time. This is not meant as a consolation, but more as a recognition that none of us can choose how much time we have left, and we need to do our best to make the most out of whatever time we have. As always, the best way to plan is to set priorities and go for them… easy to say, hard to do.

If there does come a time when the later stage of disease is reached, it is critical to know about two resources. First, there are physicians available called **palliative care specialists**. Not all patients or doctors know about what these doctors do. Palliative care doctors work to prevent and alleviate suffering, and in fact they treat anyone at any stage of a variety of illnesses. Most commonly, though, these doctors are associated with caring for patients with cancer, and typically are consulted toward the later stages of disease. They work with your oncologist or other doctors to address emotional and physical pain, they can help your loved ones to find emotional and spiritual comfort, and typically they take a holistic approach to healing the patient and the family. Please ask about a referral to a palliative care specialist in the event that you or your family is suffering, particularly if a cure is not in reach. Don't wait too long to ask about this type of referral; it is best to get ahead of issues that patients face in the later stages of their disease so that there is time for these doctors to help.

The second resource is **hospice care.** Most every oncologist has extensive experience with having patients receive this very specialized type of assistance. Depending on the circumstances, hospice care can be administered in the home or in an inpatient setting, and it is administered by highly skilled, medically-trained caregivers whose mission is to make the final months, weeks, or days as calm, dignified, pain-free, and peaceful as possible. It is amazing how, in many cases, these caring and dedicated practitioners can help a patient and their family achieve a healing transition as the patient passes. Here, too, timing matters. It is best to discuss with your doctor how and when to think about hospice care.

CHAPTER 6

Pain Management

How should I deal with pain?

Talk about it. Ask your doctor about it and talk to your care partner about your concerns. Ask what to expect from tests and from the disease process, and realize that all patients react to pain and pain medication differently. Pain and other discomforts might plague some patients continuously, but for many pain is temporary and manageable. Other patients may feel no pain at all during their entire course of treatment.

Manage anxiety about pain. Many patients have anxiety about pain and about taking pain medication. Properly dealing with this anxiety can actually help you control your reaction to pain. Managing anxiety starts with talking to you doctor. Of course, counseling and anxiety medication can be appropriate in some cases. But, if you have anxiety about pain or how to treat it, start by discussing your feelings with your doctor. Though some patients are reluctant to try pain medication, it's impossible to know how it will affect you unless you take it. Many times your main cancer doctor is more than capable of helping you to manage pain effectively. However, your doctor can send you to a pain management specialist if needed.

Treat the pain early. If possible, get pain medication into your system either just as the pain is starting, or, in cases of chronic pain or situations where you know pain can be expected, even *before* the pain begins. As with most health issues, when it comes to pain, prevention is better than cure. Studies show taking medication earlier in the "pain curve" actually reduces the amount of medication necessary to manage pain effectively.

Over time, patients may become tolerant of narcotics, which essentially means that their bodies get used to the medication and stop responding as well as they used to. For most, a simple increase in dose should take care of this, but it may be challenging to get to a therapeutic dose without getting side effects such as sleepiness or, in rare cases, a decrease in breathing, which can be dangerous. Tolerance is not the same thing as dependence or addiction (the psychological or physiological need for medication).

Most patients don't want to take any medications that they do not have to take. In general, this is a healthy attitude, but too many cancer patients fear pain medication. For most, dependence and addiction do not need to be major concerns. Among the types of medication that patients are typically concerned about are narcotics, but many types of pain medication exist, as well as alternative therapies such as acupuncture.

Narcotics are often a good choice. Some patients do not get any sensorial depression (meaning they don't get groggy) if they have pain and take the correct dose of narcotics. However, if that same patient takes the same dose a few days later when they are out of pain, they will indeed get a bit sleepy.

In some cases patients may feel "out of it", even without having taken enough medicine to manage the pain. Patients react to pain medications differently. The right dosage for optimum pain management will vary depending on how the patient's body reacts to the specific medication, among other things. That's why it is important to try pain medication, so that you can gauge your individual reaction. Of course while taking pain medication, you should not drive, operate heavy equipment, or engage in any activity where grogginess might harm you or others until you discuss that activity with the doctor who is prescribing the medication.

Some people worry that taking pain medication signifies weakness or that their cancer is progressing. Certainly taking pain medication does not mean that you are a weak person. Furthermore, no decent person would stigmatize a patient with cancer for taking pain medication. In some cases, pain does signify cancer progression, but not always. Pain medication is just one more tool to help you get back to what is important in life.

There are cases where patients become "dependent" on pain medication, which generally means that they have a psychological need to take pain medication to feel good from day to day. Sometimes when a disease causes chronic pain, the patient is in fact dependent on the pain medication to treat the pain. However, many people worry that they will be dependent on the medication even if they do not feel pain, and this rarely happens.

For some patients, but fortunately very few, physical and psychological dependence or addiction does occur. In most cases, these effects can be broken by a slow process of gradually lowering the dose of narcotics, which should only be done under a doctor's supervision for safety reasons. However, there is no specific test that says one person is dependent or addicted and another is not. This may sound scary, but usually the best thing for patients is to go ahead with taking the pain medication, and by experience they will determine the best way to use this tool for their personal situation.

Some patients find themselves working with a

doctor who undertreats their pain. The first way to guard against this is—you guessed it—to communicate with your doctor and care partner. Let them know what you need. If your doctor is reluctant to address your needs, ask why. Most doctors respond well to a heartfelt talk. If you find this is not the case with your doctor, then you may need to find a doctor who is able to treat all aspects of your specific condition.

A patient who has a past or present addiction needs to address the subject honestly with his or her doctor, care partner, and other addiction support mechanisms that might be in place. An established or former addiction creates a difficult situation that cannot be fully addressed in this book beyond saying that, as always, communication is key.

In some situations your doctor might send you to a pain management specialist. Like other physicians, these folks are caring practitioners, but they typically focus mainly on managing physical pain, and may not have a holistic approach to help with other issues. The second specialty is the palliative care specialist. Palliative care specialists, which we discussed at the end of Chapter 5 (see above), focus on physical and emotional pain, and also have a holistic approach to helping entire families to heal.

NOTES

CHAPTER 7

Clinical Trials

Do I qualify to participate in a clinical trial?

If you have a cancer curable through conventional methods, you likely will not need a **clinical trial** (also called a clinical protocol), although you still might want to consider participating in one. For those whose cancer is not curable through conventional methods, qualifying for a clinical trial can be a big advantage, because clinical trials provide options, and options are good!

There are many good reasons to participate in a clinical trial:

1. You might directly benefit from the therapy. However, this is not true for all trials. This issue is discussed as part of the informed consent process, when the doctor running the trial goes over the potential benefits and risks.

2. Others might benefit from your participation.

3. You will likely get even more attentive medical care. Most clinical trial participants have their medical condition followed very closely by doctors and nurses as part of the trial protocol.

4. You might get study medication at no cost to you.

5. You might be able to get a medication that you would not be able to get without participating in the trial.

Of course there are potential risks that you should consider, and the study coordinator and doctor running the trial will discuss these with you and give you a chance to ask questions.

You might ask, "Will I be a guinea pig?" That is a common question, but the specific concerns that engender the question are what should be discussed. There are many types of clinical trials. Some are observational, meaning that you will not be given any therapy. Your condition will only be observed in order to advance the understanding of your disease or its treatment.

In other clinical trials participants are randomly assigned to receive either one type of therapy or another type. So for example, if 100 people enroll in the trial, 50 will be randomly assigned to receive Approach A and 50 will be assigned to receive Approach B. Therefore, if you choose to participate, you will have a 50 percent chance (like flipping a coin) of receiving one therapy or the other. Usually this is a double-blind process, meaning that neither the doctors running the trial nor the participants know which therapy they are receiving; they only know that they have been randomly assigned to receive one or the other. It is extremely important to make trials blinded since without blinding, bias can be introduced. If the participants or their doctors know which arm they are randomized to, it is very common for them to feel it working even if it is not effective. Similarly, if the study is not blinded an adverse reaction might either be ignored or inappropriately attributed to the experimental therapy.

Of course, even in double blinded trials, some study personnel who are not involved in administering the treatment are aware of which patients are receiving which therapy. These might include a safety monitoring board (SMB) comprised of physicians and other personnel that meet at pre-determined times throughout the trial to make sure it is safe to continue. In addition, the SMB can meet on an as needed basis if safety concerns arise. Sometimes the SMB stops a trial early because they discover an unacceptably serious adverse reaction, and/or if the therapy is truly not working. However, sometimes a study is stopped early if the therapy is working better than expected and no further investigation is needed. This is typically a very desirable situation where the therapy that was effective is often then offered to everyone.

In some active-controlled clinical trials, the "standard of care" therapy (the one that is typically used in clinical practice) is compared to an experimental therapy or to a combination of standard plus experimental therapy. In other words, both treatment arms receive active medication. This often makes participants feel better, because they know they will be receiving some sort of therapy no matter which treatment arm they are assigned to.

However, some clinical trials are placebo-controlled. This means that you might be randomly assigned to receive the experimental medication or to receive a dummy substance, such as a "sugar pill". Placebo-controlled trials are typically done when there is no therapy for a particular clinical situation. In such cases, it is perfectly ethical, and indeed important, to include a placebo arm, since in that particular clinical situation doctors are not sure whether the experimental therapy will help or harm the person taking it.

So are participants in clinical trials "guinea pigs?" No. They are fully informed of the known risks and benefits of participation (though these are usually not completely known for experimental therapies). Trial participants are integral partners in our search for new and better therapies. There really is no way to figure out if a therapy works without designing a rigorous clinical trial that tries to eliminate bias. Moreover, the doctors that are clinical trial investigators are usually among the best and brightest. Medicine is their passion; chances are they want to find a cure almost as much as you do. They really do not want to hurt anyone, and they want you to be comfortable with any decisions that are made.

In addition, there are a series of safeguards that are designed to protect you. First, the Department of Health and Human Services (HHS), a federal cabinet-level department that oversees, among other things, the Office for Human Research Protections (OHRP) that governs institutional review boards (IRBs) that review and approve clinical trial protocols and informed consent documents.

The entity that funds a clinical trial (the sponsor) and the physicians who will run the trial must submit their study protocols and informed consent documents to be evaluated by an IRB. These boards are typically composed of a combination of physicians, laypersons, attorneys, and ethicists who work together to make sure that clinical trials are reasonably safe, and that the informed consent documents are clear and appropriate. For very serious diseases that have no known treatments, the IRBs are often more accepting of riskier therapies as long as the risks are clearly disclosed.

IRBs review at least two documents, the study protocol and the informed consent form. The study protocol discusses the study procedures as well as the criteria that outline which patients are eligible, or ineligible, to participate. The informed consent form outlines the study procedures for participants: the possible benefits and risks, inclusion/exclusion criteria, and important contacts, such as the study coordinator (the person you should contact if you are considering participating in the trial) and the doctor running the trial. The informed consent form is supposed to be written in straightforward language that someone in elementary school could understand.

Moreover, there are protected groups, such as children, prison inmates, and mentally challenged individuals, for whom special safeguards are in place. Participation in the clinical trial is always voluntary, and you can discontinue participation for any reason. Your medical care and attention from doctors and nurses must not be adversely affected whether you choose to participate in a clinical trial or not, or whether you drop out of the trial. You should never feel coerced into participating. If you choose to participate in a clinical trial, you must sign the informed consent form in order to give your permission to be enrolled into the study.

As discussed above, there is usually an independent data safety monitoring board (or data monitoring committee) that monitors the ongoing trial to determine whether the trial should be stopped early either because the risks are too high (too many participants are experiencing adverse events) or because the experimental therapy is so effective that further study is not needed. The next level of protection comes from the study coordinator and the physician running the trial. Many trials are carried out at multiple treatment centers simultaneously. The study coordinator and doctor that you will see may be one of many throughout the country. It's truly important that you trust them and that they are thoughtful about whether it is in your best interest to participate. Obviously, you make that decision together with them, but that brings us to your final level of protection—*you* and your care partner. Make sure your best judgment is telling you that participating in the clinical trial is your best option.

The decision about whether or not to participate in a clinical trial should be considered with the same care you give to all your other treatment decisions—it's even best to use a similar approach, though some minor differences do exist.

1. Determine if you qualify to participate. Clinical trials have specific entry, or "inclusion" criteria that say you are eligible to participate and specific "exclusion" criteria that disqualify your participation. The study coordinator will evaluate your case closely to determine whether you are able to participate.

2. As with all your other treatment decisions, you and your doctor should ask: "What are the treatment goals?" Determine what the clinical trial is *realistically* designed to accomplish: total cure, longer life, increased disease-free survival, improvement of symptoms. Decide if the trial's goals are aligned with your goals.

3. If you qualify for a clinical trial, you might have two options: to continue with standard therapy, or participate in the clinical trial. However, it may be that participating in a clinical trial is your *only* treatment option. The key question at this point is how much risk to assume, and there is no easy answer to this question. Talk about this with your doctor and care partner.

How do I find out about clinical trials?

There is not always a clear path to this information, but the Internet is making it much easier. Your doctor is a good place to start, as well as other patients, support groups, or the Internet (see *Chapter 8: The Internet and Other Resources* for a more in-depth discussion of this).

Who sponsors (pays for and runs) clinical trials?

Typically clinical trials are paid for by the **National Institutes of Health** (NIH) using taxpayer money or a pharmaceutical or biotechnology company. In other instances individual institutions or doctors pay for clinical trials through private funds from hospitals, patient advocacy groups, private donations, etc. The trials are typically administered either at an academic medical center (one affiliated with a medical school), a private medical center, or an individual doctor's office. Ultimately, the results are reported to whichever entity pays for the trial, and often to the FDA, which has many functions, one of which is regulating and monitoring clinical trials.

NOTES

112

CHAPTER 8

The Internet and Other Resources

How should I research cancer using the Internet?

First, understand your goals. Like your doctor, your mind, and your medical therapy, the Internet is just a tool: a powerful tool, yes, but one that most of us use unsupervised. Chances are very good that you'll be doing your Internet research alone, with family, or with friends. If you delay your research until after you have definitively been diagnosed with cancer and have had your first visit with your cancer doctor, you can likely work more effectively. However, you might feel better if you search before you know exactly what is going on with your health. Either way, follow these three simple rules:

Rule 1: Explore at your own risk

There are risks to exploring the Internet. The most common risk is to your psyche in terms of feeling unnecessary or misguided emotions. The second risk is getting inaccurate information that could lead to making poor decisions. The third risk is being victimized by a scam that preys on your need to feel hopeful. Be careful. Verify information with your doctor before you act on it. With experience, you can effectively use the Internet to maximize your knowledge about cancer; however, you will likely need to bring any information about novel or experimental treatments to your care team to help you evaluate it.

Rule 2: Define your questions *before* you search

Do you want to know how long you have to live? Chances are if you try to answer this question by searching the Internet, the information that you obtain will almost certainly not apply exactly to you. Many of us assume that, critical illness or not, we are going to beat the odds and live until we're 100+ years old.

Internet research into pancreatic cancer (particularly of the adenocarcinoma type) will inform you that the prospect of surviving more than a year is likely doubtful. It will also inform you that life expectancy with papillary thyroid cancer might be close to normal, provided you have a small tumor that has not spread beyond the thyroid gland.

While both pieces of information are generally true, there are always exceptions: *Some* patients with pancreatic cancer are still alive 20 years after diagnosis, and *some* patients with thyroid cancer will die within a year. The bottom line is that regarding tumors with very bad or very good prognoses, trusted sites on the Internet will be reasonably accurate sources of information for most, *but not all* patients. The diagnoses and prognoses of most patients with cancer fall somewhere in the middle of the spectrum.

Your best, easiest, most accurate method of understanding your diagnosis and prognosis is to schedule an appointment with your doctor to discuss it. If you're trying to prepare yourself for news about your specific condition, the Internet is typically not particularly useful, because your particular outcome is so dependent on your specific medical circumstances. However, there are ways the Internet can complement other resources, and these fall into three categories.

First, if you're researching general or specific information that you plan to verify later with your doctor or nurse, particularly information about how to deal with having procedures or treatments, the Internet can be very helpful. Your doctor's office might be a well-run clinical operation and have most procedures standardized, but there is no way that they will think of everything. Should you premedicate with anti-emetics (anti-nausea medications) before having chemotherapy? What types of radiation therapies are used for prostate cancer and how will they affect sexual function? Gather this type of information to identify issues and supplement what your doctor or nurse has told you, and then you can verify the information with them.

Second, information about novel or experimental therapies, including names of experimental medication as well as clinical trials and which centers are doing them, can be found on the Internet. Indeed, the amount of information about experimental therapies and clinical trials can be overwhelming, even for medical professionals. The best approach is to first understand your own disease and condition, then try to determine which, if any, of the clinical trials being run apply to patients with the particular type and stage of cancer you have, who also share your specific circumstances. Many trials apply to patients with very specific clinical circumstances, such as patients with metastatic breast cancer who have already completed at least two different chemotherapy regimens. Again, you will need help from your doctor to verify what you have found, but the Internet can be useful to research emerging therapies.

Third, the Internet can be indispensable if you want to get the "word on the street." News sites can be useful, but keep in mind their business model is to sell advertising, and to do this they must attract and keep eyeballs on the page (see below for how to use the news). Blogs are written by individuals discussing a topic; though they can be useful, they can also be treacherous. Some blogs promote rumors and spread inaccurate information. However, people are often quite candid online, particularly if they feel anonymous. Sometimes blogs can provide information, particularly about others' experiences, that you cannot obtain by any other means. Let me repeat that all information must be verified by credible sources, including your doctor. As in so many aspects of life, in our collective fight against cancer, the Internet will continue to fundamentally change the ways in which we connect with each other, and will expand our ability to obtain at and promote the truth. It is especially important to follow Rule 1 if you decide to read blogs about cancer or if you feel like perusing the news.

Social media and cancer advocacy groups now have so many resources comprised of interested, engaged individuals dedicated to helping individuals undergoing cancer treatment and cancer survivors. They can be a great place to get "virtual" though very real support. That said, remember, they are populated mostly by lay persons, many of whom are quite opinionated, and who may, however unintentionally, espouse inaccurate and misleading information. Becoming active members on these sites can be helpful, but doing so requires extra caution.

Rule 3: Know where to start your search before you begin.

I have found the following websites useful, reliable sources of accurate information. Of course, many other websites, particularly those run by medical societies and organizations dedicated to specific types of cancer, can be extremely valuable. In addition, various institutions, including the one where you are being evaluated and treated, might be incredibly helpful to you for many reasons. But by starting with these sites, you will begin with some of the most comprehensive and trusted cancer websites, which, in turn, might direct you to other reputable websites that deal with your specific cancer.

www.cancer.net

The American Society of Clinical Oncology (ASCO), a major medical society for cancer doctors, set up this website to provide information and address the concerns of patients with cancer and cancer survivors. It's a well-designed, logically organized site with some great links to other informative sites and resources for specific types of cancers and cutting-edge research.

www.cancer.org

This is the website for the American Cancer Society (ACS), a not-for-profit organization supported by donors. The site offers easily accessible information and resources about cancer information, statistics, prevention, and survivorship issues. In addition, ACS publishes important guidelines on cancer prevention and cancer care, and sponsors grant programs that fund cutting-edge research.

www.cancer.gov

This is the website for the National Cancer Institute (NCI), which is part of the NIH. This expansive site has gotten much more user-friendly over the past few years. It is a comprehensive source of disease information, cancer clinical trials, and government policy on cancer.

www.livestrong.org

This is the Livestrong Foundation website. It provides information and important support resources available to those dealing with cancer. This is a great site for cancer survivorship and advocacy, and provides many ways to become active in the fight against cancer.

www.aacr.org

The American Association for Cancer Research (AACR) is a major cancer research-focused medical society. The site provides a great deal of clinical information and resources for patient, survivors, and advocates.

www.clinicaltrials.gov

This website lists *all* types of clinical trials available, not just those for cancer. It is searchable based on multiple criteria, so it really helps if you understand your particular condition, including the stage of your tumor and overall medical situation.

www.nccn.com

This is an incredibly valuable site devoted to patients, caregivers, and their families. It offers a wealth of information about patient care guidelines, how to manage transition from hospital to home, how to care for patients at home, and life after cancer. The parent site, www.nccn.org, has authoritative guidelines that many physicians look to when deciding which care to provide to specific patients with specific tumor types at each stage of disease.

How do I best use news about cancer?

Do not believe everything that you read or see. Even the most credible news sources often tell only part of the story. Of course the medical community has made many important advances recently, and many of these advances have been in the news. However, if a complete cure for a common cancer type were really imminent, it would likely not be one random story buried in an obscure website. If you are seeing information on a major network or Internet news site, it is quite possible that the true story:

1. Has many more positive and negative aspects that are not being communicated to you.

2. Is a muted version of what you are seeing and hearing. In other words, the story is either not as exciting as is being portrayed if it is about a breakthrough, or not as bad if it is a story about a potential risk. Of course, some information is truly exciting and some represents a truly needed warning. Again, it's best to make your doctor aware of the information and ask for his or her opinion.

NOTES

122

CHAPTER 9

Cancer Prevention

If you are reading this book, you may already have been diagnosed with cancer. Reading about prevention might seem like "shutting the barn door after the horse is gone." But is it? Absolutely not. First, people are living longer than ever with cancer. It's not unheard of for people living with cancer to develop one or more other types of cancer as well. Learning how to prevent another form of cancer while you're fighting the first could be life-saving information for you. Also, you can use your unique position as a person who has confronted cancer to advocate for cancer prevention for those around you. Even if you are not a cancer activist on a national stage, you can become an incredibly effective advocate within your direct sphere of influence. Many people will listen.

Tobacco use is associated with an increase in at least ten types of cancer. Let's consider how this might work. In smokers, the mouth, trachea (wind pipe), and lungs are directly exposed to tobacco smoke, and the lungs can absorb toxins into the bloodstream, which circulates throughout the body.

At night we swallow the fluid that is produced in our mouth and lungs. If the fluid we swallow contains tobacco toxins, the organs of our gastrointestinal (GI) tract (mouth, esophagus, stomach, small intestine, colon, rectum, and anus) are exposed to those toxins. Our GI tract absorbs the toxins, which filter through the liver—poisoning it in the process—and then enter the bloodstream. Some of the toxins are then excreted through the kidneys, into the bladder, and out through the urethra, exposing all these organs to the tobacco toxins as well. That's a substantial number of organs potentially exposed to tobacco toxins.

It's no surprise then that in America, if people stopped using *all* tobacco products, including cigarettes, cigars, pipes, and smokeless tobacco, based on one estimate there would be approximately one-third fewer cancer deaths (Department of Health and Human Services, 2004). That means that *each year* in the U.S., 170,000 or more people could be spared dying of cancer.

Some cancers start as a **precancerous** condition that can be detected by a screening test. One of the best examples is the identification of a polyp that can be removed at the time of a colonoscopy, thus decreasing the risk of developing colon cancer. Most of the more than 150,000 colon and rectal cancers diagnosed in America each year could be prevented by early detection and removal of precancerous polyps. Indeed, the incidence of colon and rectal cancers has been decreasing steadily since the institution of colonoscopy screening guidelines. You should discuss your risk of colon cancer with your doctor and find out when you should get a colonoscopy.

Screening for breast cancer is effective. Since precancerous breast cancer abnormalities are harder to detect, screening is aimed at detecting breast cancer at an early stage. Though controversy exists regarding how and when to screen for breast cancer, everyone would agree that women should periodically examine their own breasts and have breast exams by their physician. Breast cancers can also be detected early using a **mammogram** or other types of imaging in some women. Of course it is best to get specific recommendations from your physician.

Similarly for men, proper application of a periodic **digital rectal exam** of the prostate, and a **prostate-specific antigen (PSA)** blood test could lead to early detection and treatment of prostate cancer. In addition, if every adolescent male and adult man performed testicular self-exams and had periodic testicular exams by a doctor, the rate of testicular cancer-related deaths would be significantly reduced.

Some cancers are caused by infectious agents. If everyone at risk were vaccinated against the Hepatitis B virus, the rate of liver cancer would decrease. Similarly, if those at risk were vaccinated against the human papilloma virus (HPV), the rate of cervical cancer would also decrease. For women, a periodic **pap smear** is another good way to check for cervical cancer or a pre-cancerous condition before it becomes cervical cancer.

Most people should avoid intentionally exposing their skin to the sun for long periods of time. Sunblock, with a minimum sun protection factor (SPF) of 15, should be used throughout life. In addition, periodic self-exams of the skin and examinations by a doctor would dramatically reduce the rate of skin cancer and help treat it earlier.

Though we are just beginning to learn about this issue, most sunscreens contain chemicals that might pose risks of their own. At this time, it seems prudent to use sunscreens that use only inorganic minerals such as zinc oxide or titanium dioxide and are designed to block the sun immediately upon application.

Though protection from large amounts of sun and from sunburn is important, exposure to sunlight is an important stimulus for the body to produce vitamin D, which is important for proper bone health and probably also for cancer prevention. As with many other topics, please discuss sun exposure with your doctor.

Though more cancers can be prevented than the types I have mentioned here, with the elimination of tobacco use, proper application of safe sun protection, vaccination against Hepatitis B and HPV, and screening checks for colon, breast, prostate, skin, cervical, and testicular cancer, we could save hundreds of thousands of lives each year.

NOTES

128

CHAPTER 10

Looking Forward

Modern medicine will continue to fulfill its promise and I believe we will eventually find a cure for all cancers, and as research continues to progress, prevent all cancers. The best way to accelerate medical breakthroughs is to come together as a society: cancer survivors and those who care about them, medical professionals, community and medical organizations, and government.

Learning how to approach the diseases we face and engage each other in ways that maintain respect and break down barriers is crucial. As we progress as individuals and as a society, we must leverage what we learn in one area of life to accelerate our advances in others. That is what I have tried to encourage in this book. I am eternally hopeful and optimistic, and I believe that through our collective human spirit we will solve our problems.

Patients today have an increasing array of choices and resources. The Internet is an incredibly powerful tool to keep the dialogue moving forward and for coordinating and organizing our efforts, and at its best—intelligently and with caution—it can facilitate a coalescence of ideas and actions. As I mentioned, it is important to use the Internet responsibly, with caution and verify information with your healthcare team. Clinical trials offer hope and options for many patients facing cancer, and translate discovery into clinically meaningful advances in diagnosis and treatment.

Many areas are advancing rapidly, including immunotherapy and biologically-targeted cancer treatments. However, one area is advancing at an incredible pace. Personalized medicine—leveraging genetic discoveries to inform individualized diagnosis and treatment of each patient—is an incredibly exciting frontier that we are already starting to use in clinical medicine. Indeed, today it is becoming more common for doctors to order laboratory tests to decode a patient's entire **genome** (the study of the entire genome is called **genomics**), and in doing so we can now know the entire sequence of all of our genes. More information is being discovered every day about how individual genes and groups of genes contribute to various diseases. Knowing our gene sequences and pairing that information with the risks associated with particular gene variants and mutations allows us to assess a person's risk of getting a particular disease *before* he or she is actually affected by it.

In addition, many variations in gene sequence are associated with efficacy and safety issues with individual medications. Though other factors besides gene sequences help determine responses to medications, the fact remains that **pharmacogenomics** is now a burgeoning field. Pharmacogenomics is beginning to explain why medications only work on certain patients, and this field allows us to predict who will respond and why, and for whom a particular medication might cause adverse effects.

Finally, we can now sequence the entire genome of a patient's tumor and compare it to the sequence of his or her normal tissues to see exactly which genes are mutated and, in some cases, figure out which of those mutated genes contributed to or caused the cancer. In some cases we can use that information to understand prognosis and more rationally choose which medications to use.

With this technology, we can now begin to answer the questions: "What went wrong to cause this cancer, and how can we best target this particular tumor?" In some cases, the therapy is itself a piece of DNA or **RNA** that is introduced into the body (**gene therapy**) and designed to inhibit or produce a particular substance.

As you might imagine, personalized medicine makes for some important ethical and practical discussions about whether and when all of this sequencing should be done. As with other emerging technologies and therapies, I am confident that we will work hard as medical practitioners and as a society to use these innovations wisely. I want to close by wishing each of you a healthier day than yesterday, and I look forward to the time when cancer is a thing of the past.

Your "CAT" is not your "PET"

A GLOSSARY TO LIVE BY

Knowing definitions of key medical terms creates a sense of familiarity with the topic of cancer, and familiarity is the first step to understanding. Understanding a daunting topic makes it less overwhelming, and thereby promotes a sense of calm. And staying calm is the key to making decisions that beat cancer! To put it more practically, the meaning of words is one of the first things children learn as they begin to communicate. Learning the definitions to these words will enhance your ability to understand your medical issues and to communicate effectively with your medical team.

Adjuvant

The term *adjuvant* refers to a second therapy that is added after a first therapy. For example, someone might have surgery followed by adjuvant chemotherapy.

Adverse Reaction (*also* Side Effect)

An ***adverse reaction*** can occur from any treatment. Treatments can have known toxicities that can be common or rare, and can vary from mild to life-threatening. Some adverse reactions are managed by reducing or skipping a dose of the therapy. More severe reactions may require admission to the hospital. You should discuss the potential toxicities and adverse reactions of your treatments with your doctor.

Benign

Benign means that a tumor or abnormal area is not cancer. Specifically, it will not metastasize (spread to another part of the body). Most benign tumors cause no significant health problems, but some can grow and become dangerous depending on their location and which structures they encroach upon.

Biological Therapy

Biological therapy (targeted therapy) is usually an injectable substance designed to mimic or target a substance in the body in order to either promote or inhibit a specific cellular function. This specificity is the main difference between biological therapy and traditional chemotherapy. Biological therapies can have side effects and only certain cancers are treated with biological therapies.

Biopsy

A *biopsy* is a sample of a tumor or abnormal area that is removed from the body and examined under a microscope or in other ways. This is done to tell whether the tissue is cancer or a different disease, as well as to determine some characteristics that will help you and your doctor know what to do about it.

Cancer Stage

Cancer stage describes how advanced a cancer is in terms of its spread throughout the body. In general, the higher the stage, the worse the prognosis.

Care Partner

A *care partner* is a person who is able to dedicate time, thoughtfulness, and emotional energy to helping you fight your disease. Sometimes it's best to have one main person in this role and utilize the other people around you for support. However, you may find it beneficial to have more than one care partner. This is not only a big job, but also one that takes organization and follow-through.

Care Plan

A *care plan* (*treatment plan*) refers to the comprehensive list of diagnostic procedures and therapies that you will have. It is vitally important to have a plan and to understand why that plan is the best one for you.

CAT (Computed Axial Tomography) or CT Scan

A *CAT* or *CT scan* is an X-ray-based test. During the scan you lie on a moving table as it slides through a large doughnut-shaped machine. An X-ray camera spins around your body as you move through the doughnut and creates images that look like slices of your body, enabling visualization of your internal organs. Patients are often given barium to drink prior to the procedure so their bowels appear white on the scans. This helps the radiologist (imaging doctor) see the difference between organs. Dye can also be administered intravenously (directly into a vein) to allow visualization of the blood vessels. Since this dye can adversely affect the kidneys, kidney function is usually checked prior to having a CAT scan.

CBC (Complete Blood Count)

A *CBC* is a blood test that measures white blood cells (infection-fighting cells), red blood cells (oxygen-carrying cells), and platelets (for clotting blood). Other measures are also listed on the CBC, but they all function to further describe aspects of these three cell types.

Cells

Cells are the basic functional units in our bodies. Our bodies contain trillions of cells that ideally work together in harmony. Nearly all cells have a limited lifespan, and are replenished on a regular basis. A cancer cell grows more rapidly than it should or resists dying, and it can detach from the main tumor and travel to other parts of the body, with the potential to grow in those other areas (metastasize).

Chemotherapy

Chemotherapy can be either a liquid medication administered into a vein or a pill taken by mouth that causes rapidly multiplying cells to die, often by targeting and disrupting their DNA. Since cancer cells can multiply more rapidly or differently than normal cells, the hope is that *only* the cancer cells will be killed. However, since normal rapidly growing cells such as hair cells, cells lining the intestines, and blood-forming cells can also be affected by chemotherapy, the side effects of hair loss, nausea and vomiting, anemia and infection can occur. Other side effects can occur depending on the particular medication and how your body reacts to it.

Chemotherapy Regimen vs. Chemotherapy Cycle

A *chemotherapy regimen* refers to a full course of chemotherapy, while a *chemotherapy cycle* is one instance of receiving chemotherapy medication. For example, a regimen may be to give three drugs together every three weeks for a total of five times. A cycle (or round) represents one administration of the drug(s). This example is a three-drug regimen that has five cycles. Many different regimens exist, and each cycle could contain the same or different drugs.

Chromosomes

Chromosomes are the structures within the cells that contain all of the genes needed for development and function of the cells. Humans have 46 chromosomes (23 pairs), each of which carries hundreds or thousands of genes. Each of us, except for identical twins, has a unique set of genes, though the actual number of bases that differ between two humans are not that numerous on a percentage basis. That explains why we all have the same parts that function in the same way, yet each of us look just a bit different and our organs have slight differences in function and disease susceptibility.

Clinical Trial

Clinical trials are usually sponsored (paid for and administered) by the National Institutes of Health (NIH), a pharmaceutical or biotechnology company, adademic institution, or a not-for-profit organization. Typically, clinical trials are studies that compare a current therapy to an experimental therapy, to the current therapy *plus* an experimental therapy or to a placebo (an inactive "sugar pill"). In *Chapter 7: Clinical Trials*, potential advantages and disadvantages of participating in a clinical trial are discussed.

Colonoscopy

During a *colonoscopy* a flexible tube with a camera at the end is inserted through the anus into the rectum and colon in order to find and remove a polyp or tumor or to diagnose a gastrointestinal condition.

Complete Response

Complete response is a term that usually applies to a clinical trial endpoint; it typically means that after a particular treatment, no tumor can be found. This is obviously a good sign, but it does not necessarily mean that the patient has been cured.

Diagnosis

A *diagnosis* is the name assigned to a disease—for example, "diabetes," "hypertension," or "colon cancer."

Digital Rectal Exam

During a *digital rectal exam*, a doctor inserts a gloved finger into the rectum to examine the size of the prostate, check other structures, or check for blood. This is an important screening test for prostate, rectal, and colon cancer.

Disease-Free Survival (*also* Relapse-Free Survival)

Disease-free survival is a term that can be used in clinical practice, but it often applies to a clinical trial endpoint. It refers to the length of time that you are alive without detectable cancer in your body after you are given a particular therapy. This does not necessarily mean that a patient is cured.

DNA (Deoxyribonucleic Acid)

DNA is composed of four types of molecular building blocks: adenine, cytosine, thymine, and guanine. Strings of these building blocks in a specific sequence make up a gene. A chromosome contains a large amount of DNA with many genes. When DNA within a cell (other than in sperm or eggs) is damaged (mutated), cancer can result. Though germ cell cancers (cancers that arise from cells that form sperm and eggs) can occur, mutations in DNA in sperm or egg cells more typically cause birth defects or predispose the offspring to cancer or other diseases.

Five-Year Survival

Five-year survival is how cancer doctors speak about the percentage of patients who are likely to beat their cancer. Many cancers come back within five years of treatment, so this is an important milestone. However, some cancers are capable of coming back much later, and five years does not necessarily mean a cure, although it might. In addition, statistics regarding five-year survival allows doctors to compare how well different treatments work and how aggressive a particular cancer is.

Food and Drug Administration (FDA)

The *FDA* is the part of the federal government and regulates, among other things, drug approvals and clinical trials. The website address is *www.fda.gov.*

Gene

A *gene* is a stretch of DNA that contains the instructions, or recipe, for how to make a particular protein or proteins. Proteins are substances that are in all of our cells and carry out essential body functions.

Gene Therapy

Gene therapy is a form of biological therapy. A piece of DNA or RNA is injected into the body. The DNA induces the production of a particular protein that either substitutes for a defective protein or targets a process within the tumor that will cause the cancer cells to die or become more susceptible to other treatments. Injected RNA can bind to DNA or RNA to regulate how and whether a gene is turned on or off.

Genetic Counselors

Genetic counselors are specialists who may not be doctors, but typically have advanced training in helping patients and families understand genetic testing. They can help to determine the risk of disease and the particular meaning of gene sequences and mutations.

Genomics

Genomics is the study of the entire genome (all the genes in the body). Knowing the gene sequences can help to assess the risk of a particular disease, know how a medication will work in that particular patient, or help to pick the right medication or therapy to treat a particular disease. Ultimately genomics will be used to prevent disease.

Hemoglobin (HGB)

Hemoglobin is a protein in the red blood cells (RBCs) that carries oxygen to tissues. Low hemoglobin or a low number of RBCs is referred to as anemia.

Hospice Care

Hospice care refers to in-home or inpatient care instituted during the final stages of disease. This type of care focuses on keeping the patient comfortable and facilitating meaningful and peaceful interactions with family and friends.

Lesion

A *lesion* is a generic term for an abnormal area that may refer to a tumor or something other than a tumor, such as a rash.

Liquid Tumor

Cancerous cells that derive from cells that normally circulate throughout our body and are not connected to each other are referred to as a *liquid tumor*. Leukemia, a cancer of blood-forming cells that floats around in your bloodstream and bone marrow, is a good example.

Lymph Nodes

Lymph nodes are like small filters containing many white blood cells through which lymph fluid flows. You may have noticed swollen glands (as they are sometimes called) in your neck when you have a cold or sinus infection. Lymph nodes are often the sites where cancer cells first collect and grow when they escape from the original tumor.

Malignant

Malignant means the tumor or abnormal area is cancerous (and has the ability to spread to other parts of the body). If a cancer is caught before it has spread, it can be cured if it is completely removed or eradicated. It is impossible to tell for sure whether a tumor has spread.

Mammogram

A *mammogram* is an X-ray-based screening test for early detection of breast cancer or suspicious breast areas that need to be biopsied.

Median Survival

Median survival is another way that doctors measure survival after diagnosis or treatment. Specifically, it is the amount of time that half of patients with a disease live. In other words, half of the patients will die before the time to median survival, and half will die after.

Metastasize (*noun* Metastasis)

Metastasize means a tumor spreads to another part of the body, such as lung cancer that has spread to the liver. In this instance, the person does not have lung cancer and liver cancer, he or she has lung cancer that has metastasized to the liver.

MRI (Magnetic Resonance Imaging)

An *MRI* is similar to a CAT scan but instead of X-rays it uses a powerful magnet to align water molecules within the body. Radio waves are then bounced off the aligned water molecules. This generates a vibration or signal. Different organs yield different signals. The MRI machine is able to detect these various signals and convert them into high-definition pictures of the inside of the body.

Mutation

An abnormality in a gene that leads to an abnormal protein is a *mutation*. Mutations are the basis of birth defects and cancer.

National Cancer Institute (NCI)

The *National Cancer Institute (NCI)* is one of

the institutes of the National Institutes of Health (NIH) and has a budget that is determined by the U.S. Congress as well as by the NIH. The NCI is responsible for setting the cancer policy for the United States. Many researchers who work at the NCI carry out cancer research. In addition, the NCI offers grants, on a competitive basis, to investigators outside of the NIH who carry out cancer research. The NCI website, *www.cancer.gov,* is a great resource for patient information, clinical trial information, and understanding new therapies.

National Institutes of Health (NIH)

The ***National Institutes of Health (NIH)*** is part of the executive branch of our federal government and is responsible for setting overall health policy as well as distributing federal research funds to doctors and scientists. The NIH is comprised of multiple institutes that focus on various areas of medicine. The website address is *www.nih.gov.*

Neoadjuvant

Neoadjuvant refers to a therapy that is given before another therapy. Often this refers to neoadjuvant radiation or chemotherapy designed to shrink a tumor to make subsequent surgical removal easier.

Oncologist

An ***oncologist*** is a doctor who specializes in cancer diagnosis and treatment.

Medical oncologist — a cancer doctor who treats patients with chemotherapy or biological therapy, and often is the main cancer doctor for the patient.

Surgical oncologist — a surgeon who specializes in treating cancer.

Radiation oncologist— a doctor who treats cancer with radiation therapy. A radiation oncologist should not be confused with a radiologist who interprets X-rays, CAT scans, and other scans.

Ostomy

An ***ostomy*** refers to a medical procedure that creates an artificial opening in the body. A colostomy is a common type of ostomy. A colostomy is sometimes needed after a colon cancer is removed. In a colostomy, a surgeon brings the proximal colon (the part that connects to the small intestine) to the abdominal wall, creating an opening. The distal part of the colon (the part that leads to the rectum and out the anus) is sewn up and remains inside the abdominal cavity. Stool that is produced by the proximal colon is collected at the colostomy opening in a sealed plastic bag and disposed of. Depending on the circumstances, the colostomy might be able to be reversed and the two ends of the colon sewn back together. Ostomies can be created in other circumstances and from other organs as well. A good website for information and resources for patients with an ostomy is *www.ostomy.org*.

Pain Management Specialist

A *pain management specialist* is a physician who has in-depth knowledge about how to approach and manage physical pain. He or she has a comprehensive understanding of the biology of pain and pain pathways in the body, as well as which medications are effective.

Palliative Care Specialist

A *palliative care specialist* is a physician who works to prevent and alleviate suffering. Though palliative care specialists can treat anyone at any stage of a variety of illnesses, most commonly these doctors are associated with caring for patients with cancer, and they typically are consulted toward the later stages of disease. They work with your oncologist or other doctors to address emotional and physical pain. They can help your loved ones to find emotional and spiritual comfort, and they typically take a holistic approach to healing patients and their families.

PAP Smear

A *Pap smear* is a screening test for cervical cancer. A doctor gently scrapes some cells from the cervix (opening of the uterus) during a pelvic exam and puts them onto a slide, which is then examined by a pathologist to determine if the cells are cancerous.

Partial Response

Partial response is a term that usually applies to a clinical trial endpoint, and the definition is typically set for that particular trial. For example, in a trial of therapy "X" compared to therapy "Y," a 25 percent reduction of tumor volume as determined by MRI scan is defined as a partial response.

Pathology Report

A *pathology report* is a document that lists the type of cancer or tumor and important features such as how aggressive the cells appear to be. The diagnosis on this report is based on tissue obtained from a biopsy that has been examined by a doctor (a pathologist) under a microscope. The information on this report doesn't tell the entire story, but it is a crucial piece of the puzzle and contains language that can be relayed from doctor to doctor. Get a copy of it and keep it for your records. Take a copy with you to each new doctor's appointment so they can put it into your chart.

Personalized Medicine

Personalized medicine can broadly mean any attempt to have medical interactions or therapy tailor-made to you. However, a popular definition these days means using genetic information (your gene sequences) to obtain a diagnostic test or administer a therapy that best fits your particular medical condition or can prevent disease in you or your relatives.

PET Scan (Positron Emission Tomography)

During a *PET scan*, a radioactive substance, for example a radioactive version of sugar, is injected into the bloodstream. Cells that are working hard or dividing fast often use more of that substance. There-fore, the radioactive substance builds up in these cells and can be detected by a large camera that detects radiation emitted from the body. The images appear as dots of different colors on a screen. A group of dots may be a tumor. Things that show up on a PET scan are often described as being "hot."

Pharmacogenomics

Pharmacogenomics refers to using genetic information (your gene sequences) to better predict whether a particular medication will be effective for you and what adverse effects might occur. In addition, this information might be used to obtain medications that best target the particular medical problem you have.

Platelets

Platelets are small structures in the blood that help the body make clots. They may be abnormally low after certain types of chemotherapy, so they are often monitored closely.

Polyp

A *polyp* is a growth often seen in the colon or rectum that may be precancerous. These can be seen and removed during a colonoscopy. Other types of polyps can arise in other organs.

Port

A *port* is a small device that is implanted under the skin, commonly on the upper chest wall. It is connected to a tube that is inserted into a large vein. The device contains a small button that can be felt under the skin into which a small needle can be inserted. This can be used as a more convenient, comfortable way of obtaining blood for lab tests or for administering chemotherapy or other medications.

Precancerous

Precancerous is a term used to define a condition that has a risk of turning into cancer. The magnitude of this risk is sometimes known for the population as a whole that has a certain condition. For example, if you have condition "X," you have a 10 percent (1 in 10) chance per year of this turning into cancer. Sometimes this risk can be reduced, and dangerous behaviors such as continued smoking, sun exposure, etc., might increase a particular risk. Some precancerous conditions can be treated or eradicated; while for others, close surveillance of your body by your physician is essential to catch the cancer at an early stage if it develops.

Prognosis

A *prognosis* is the predicted outcome of a disease, condition, or cancer. It might be described with specific data such as five-year survival, but also may be stated simply as "good" or "bad." Yet another meaning: How long a person has to live.

Prostate-Specific Antigen (PSA)

PSA is a protein produced by normal prostate cells as well as prostate cancer cells, and can be detected by a blood test. This can be used as a screening test: The higher the level, the more likely the man has prostate cancer. The PSA level can also be used to follow the response of prostate cancer to treatment and to help determine whether prostate cancer has come back after treatment.

Protein

A *protein* is made up of a string of amino acids and can serve many functions in the body from adding structure to a cell, to enzyme activity, to promoting cell growth and other functions. DNA is transcribed into RNA, which is translated into protein.

Radiation Therapy (*also* Radiotherapy)

Radiation therapy is a type of treatment designed to expose tumor cells to radiation (radioactive energy) either from an external source, such as a machine that generates radiation and can be pointed at the body, or from a radioactive material that can be implanted or injected into the body.

Red Blood Cells (RBC)

Red blood cells contain hemoglobin and carry oxygen to tissues throughout the body. Low RBCs or hemoglobin is termed anemia. Anemia can be a side effect of medications used to treat cancer or of the cancer itself.

Relapse

A *relapse* is a situation where a tumor, thought to have been eradicated, returns.

RNA (Ribonucleic Acid)

DNA is transcribed into *RNA*, which is then translated into protein. Similar to DNA, RNA is composed of four types of molecular building blocks. For RNA the building blocks are adenine, cytosine, uracil, and guanine.

Screening Test

A s*creening test* usually refers to a test that is designed to detect cancer before you have symptoms or signs, possibly as a precancerous condition.

Signs

Signs are changes in your body that you, your doctor, or others can observe. A lump that can be palpated (felt with the hands) is a sign.

Solid Tumor

A collection of abnormal cells that are connected to each other is a *solid tumor*. Most cancers are solid tumors. When some of those cells break off from the main tumor and travel throughout the body and implant in a lymph node or distant organ, the cancer is said to have metastasized.

Stem Cells

Each tissue possesses somatic *stem cells*—specialized cells that are responsible for regenerating that particular tissue. Stem cells can divide and are used by the body to replace mature cells, which typically cannot divide and are often lost or die off naturally. Cancer is thought to form from stem cells, or other less mature cells, that carry mutations in their DNA. You may have heard quite a bit about fetal and somatic stem cells as a potential cure for cancer or other diseases. This represents an active area of research.

Symptoms

Symptoms are changes in your body that only you can sense and describe to your doctor, such as pain, nausea, or fatigue.

Tumor

A *tumor* is an abnormal growth. This might also be called a nodule, shadow, neoplasm (new growth), spot, or lesion. To make matters more complex, a lesion is a generic term that may mean something other than a tumor, such as a rash. Not all tumors are cancer and not all cancers are tumors.

Ultrasound (*also* **Sonogram**)

An ***ultrasound*** is a test using a probe that sends out radio waves similar to a radar gun. These waves reflect back to the probe at different rates depending on the type of organ that they hit. The reflected radio waves are detected by the machine and translated into an image. This is the same type of test used to see a baby as it develops within the uterus, and it can be used to detect some types of cancer.

White Blood Cells (WBC)

White blood cells are cells in the blood that help fight infection and cancer. The white blood cell count may be high because of infection or inflammation or it can be low after chemotherapy. Doctors follow white blood cell counts closely.

GLOSSARY

About the Author

Dr. Pinzone is currently CEO & Medical Director of Amai, an Innovative Medical and Wellness Practice, Inc. (www.medamai.com), and Assistant Clinical Professor of Medicine at the David Geffen School of Medicine at UCLA.

Dr. Pinzone completed his medical degree at New York University School of Medicine, followed by internship and residency in Internal Medicine at Columbia-Presbyterian Medical Center. He then completed a fellowship in Endocrinology, Diabetes & Metabolism at Massachusetts General Hospital and Harvard University, where he achieved a National Research Service Award from the National Institutes of Health (NIH) to pursue molecular research on pituitary tumors.

After fellowship, Dr. Pinzone joined the faculty of The George Washington University School of Medicine, where he practiced and taught endocrinology and internal medicine and secured an NIH research grant to study the molecular biology of genes that may cause breast cancer, as well as why breast cancer metastasizes to bone. In addition, while on faculty at GW, he also studied business and graduated with a Master of Business Administration with honors.

Dr. Pinzone then joined the faculty of The Ohio State University College of Medicine where his clinical work focused on patients with diseases of the pituitary. He taught both internal medicine and endocrinology as well as continued his breast cancer research.

Dr. Pinzone was then recruited to Amgen, Inc. where he was Clinical Research Medical Director. He worked in both the Hematology/Oncology and Bone therapeutic areas. His work focused on denosumab, an antibody that inactivates RANK ligand, a naturally occurring protein that promotes bone resorption. Denosumab is used to treat patients with bone metastases from cancer as well as those with osteoporosis.

Dr. Pinzone has published multiple scientific papers, mentored many young research students and scientists, and taught medical students and doctors at all levels. He is a Fellow of the American College of Physicians and a member of Mensa. Dr. Pinzone lives in Southern California with his wife and two children.

NOTES

NOTES